Badminton Today

Badminton Today

Tariq Wadood
National Singles and Mixed Doubles Champion
Coach, National Men's and Women's Teams
Pro, Manhattan Beach Badminton Club
Manhattan Beach, CA

Karlyne Tan
Chairperson, Women's Physical Education Department
Los Angeles Valley College

Robert J. O'Connor
Series Editor for West's Physical Activities Series
Los Angeles Pierce College

West Publishing Company
St. Paul   New York   Los Angeles   San Francisco

Cover Photo: David Hanover Photography
Text Photos: David Hanover Photography
Composition: Patti Zeman
Electronic Production/ Graphics: Miyake Illustration & Design

COPYRIGHT © 1990 By WEST PUBLISHING COMPANY
50 W. Kellogg Boulevard
P.O. Box 64526
St. Paul, MN 55164-1003

All rights reserved

Printed in the United States of America

97 96 95 94 93 92 91 90   8 7 6 5 4 3 2 1 0

Library of Congress Cataloging-in-Publication Data

Wadood, Tariq.
 Badminton Today/Tariq Wadood, Karlyne Tan, Robert J. O'Connor.
 p. cm.—(West's physical activities series)
 ISBN 0-314-47596-6
 1. Badminton (Game) I. Tan, Karlyne, II. O'Connor, Robert J. III. Title.
IV. Series.
GV1007.W33 1990   89-39916
796.34 5—dc20   CIP

Table of Contents

	Foreword	ix
	Preface	xi
Chapter 1	**Introduction to Badminton**	1

Benefits of Playing Badminton 2
History of Badminton 3
Where to Play Badminton 3
Checklist on the Basics of the Game 4
Summary 4

Chapter 2	**Equipment and Facilities**	5

The Racket 6
The Shuttlecock 7
Clothing 8
Shoes 8
Socks 8
Sweatbands 8
The Court 8
Checklist for Game or Practice Equipment 10
Summary 10

Chapter 3	**Laws and Courtesies of the Game**	11

Courtesies 12
Simplified Laws (Rules) of Badminton 13
Checklist for Serving Faults 16
Summary 17

Chapter 4	**Grips, Footwork, and the Ready Position**	19

Grips 20
  Forehand Grip 20
  Backhand Grip 20
  Frying-Pan Grip 22
Checklist for the Forehand Grip 23
Checklist for the Backhand Grip 23
The Ready Position 23
  Rally Ready 23
  Ready Position for Return of Service 23
Home Base for Singles Games 24
Checklist for the Ready Position 25
Footwork 27
Warming Up 28
Checklist for the Warm-Up 31
Cooling Down 31
Summary 31

TABLE OF CONTENTS

Chapter 5	**Service and Service Return**	33

    The Serve 34
        High, Deep Serve 34
    Checklist for the High, Deep Serve 36
        Short Serve 36
    Checklist for the Low, Short Serve 38
        Flick Serve 38
        Drive Serve 38
        Backhand Serve 40
    Checklist for Low, Backhand Serve 41
    Service Return 42
        Singles Returns 42
        Doubles Returns 44
    Serving and Scoring 47
    Summary 48

Chapter 6	**Overhead Strokes**	49

    Forehand Overhead Clear 51
    Checklist for High Clear Shot 52
    Throwing Drill for Beginners 53
    Backhand Overhead Clear 54
    Attacking Clear 55
    Smash 55
    Checklist for the Smash 57
    Half-Smash 58
    Drop Shot 59
    Checklist for Drop Shot 60
    Push or Dab Shot 61
    Drive Shot 61
    Round-the-Head Shot 63
    Summary 64

Chapter 7	**Underhand Strokes and Smash Returns**	65

    Forehand Underhand Clear 66
    Backhand Underhand Clear 67
    Checklist for the Underhand Clear 68
    Underhand Drop 68
    Defensing the Smash 68
    Hairpin Drop or Dribble 69
    Checklist for the Hairpin Drop 71
    Summary 71

Chapter 8	**Strategy**	73

    Basic Strategy 74
    Your Fundamental Shots 74
    Developing Game Strategy During Warm-Up 74
    Singles Strategy 75
        Singles Serving 75
        Return of Service for Singles 75
        Singles Rally Strategy 76

Checklist for Singles Strategy   76
Doubles Strategy   78
   Doubles Serving   78
   Return of Service for Doubles   78
   Defensive Strategy for Doubles   79
   Offensive Strategy for Doubles   81
   Combination Strategy   82
Checklist for Doubles Strategy   84
Mixed Doubles Strategy   84
   Mixed Doubles Serving   84
   Return of Service for Mixed Doubles   85
   Mixed Doubles Play   85
Checklist for Mixed Doubles Strategy   86
Summary   87

Chapter 9   Drills   89

Drills   90
  1. Serving Drills   90
  2. High Service Return Drills   90
  3. Low Service Return Drills   90
  4. Straight Clear   90
  5. Crosscourt Clear   90
  6. Combination Down-the-Line and Crosscourt Clears   91
  7. Overhead Clear-and-Drop Combination   91
  8. Smash Drill   92
  9. Smash-and-Block Drill   92
 10. Smash-and-Halfcourt Drive   92
 11. Drives   92
 12. Drops   94
 13. Alternating Drops   94
 14. Overhead Drop and Underhand Clear   94
 15. Net Shots   94
 16. Quickness Drill   94
 17. Clear, Smash, Drop, Clear   96
 18. Doubles Drill   96
Self-Tests   96
  1. Deep Singles Serves   97
  2. Low Doubles Serve   97
  3. Forehand and Backhand Clears   97
  4. Drop Shots   98
  5. Smash   98
Summary   99

Chapter 10   Increasing Your Mental and Physical Potentials   101

Setting Goals   102
Mental Practice   102
   Imagery or Visualization   102
   Relaxation   103
Checklist for Learning to Relax   103
   Concentration   104

TABLE OF CONTENTS

       Physical Conditioning   104
          Strength   104
          Flexibility   108
          Aerobic (Cardiovascular) Conditioning   110
       Summary   110

Appendix A   **Laws of Badminton**   **113**
                    Laws   113
                    Appendices to the Laws of Badminton   125

Appendix B   **The United States Badminton Association**   **139**
                    Function   139
                    Activities Sponsored   139
                    Publication   139
                    Membership   140

Appendix C   **Tournament Operation**   **141**
                    Match Scheduling   141
                    The Draw   142
                    Regulations for Seeding the Draw   144
                    Some Hints on Doing the Draw   147

Appendix D   **Badminton Clubs in the United States**   **149**

                  Glossary   **153**

                  Index   **157**

Foreword

In my opinion, Tariq Wadood is one of the smoothest badminton players I have ever seen in action. This, of course, is a sign of countless hours of practice, plus a natural athletic ability which allows him to catch on quickly and execute strokes in an apparently effortless manner. For many years this has made Tariq one of the top badminton players in the world.

The combination of Tariq's skill and knowledge as a player and coach, and Karlyne Tan's excellent teaching abilities has produced an outstanding textbook on badminton. The many step-by-step photographs of our junior champions in action, in addition to concise drawings of court targets and shuttle trajectories combine to give an easy-to-read, yet comprehensive guide to playing badminton.

Those persons who study the fundamentals and strategies advocated by Tariq and Karlyne will find that their games will improve considerably. So onward to playing and enjoying this great game.

Raymond G. Scott
Executive Director
United States Badminton Association

Preface

Badminton has long had stature as a major sport in much of the world. Today, with badminton being not only an Olympic sport but also an NCAA sport, its popularity is rising rapidly in this country. With the rapid increase in the popularity of the sport we felt that it was necessary to develop a book which will allow everyone to learn the sport correctly and to enjoy it more.

The authors have worked diligently to give you the basics in every area—from the rules and courtesies of the game to the strokes and strategies. The book allows the player to progress from beginning, to intermediate, and to the advanced levels of play.

The publishers have spared no expense in allowing us to show every aspect of the game in photographs and drawings so that you readers can get the most from our presentation. We have not only explained the details of the game but we have emphasized them in various checklists in each chapter. These checklists will help you to follow a skill simply so that you can do it correctly even if you are a beginning level player.

We have not only given you more on fundamentals and strategy, we have also addressed proper conditioning—from weight training and stretching to aerobic workouts. We have also added a chapter on the mental aspects of the sport and how you can improve your game by mastering your mind's power.

We hope that you will enjoy reading the book and playing the game as much as we have enjoyed writing it for you. Have fun!

Acknowledgements

The development of this text could not have progressed without the helpful criticisms and suggestions from our colleagues. The authors gratefully acknowledge the following:

Jack Amann
Mankato State University

Patti Barrett
Southwest Texas State University

Carole A. Beeton
Diablo Valley College

Marjorie Cote
California State University, Long Beach

Jenny Feriera
Orange Coast College

Marvin R. Gray
Ball State University

Jerry Isom
Miami-Dade Community College

Pat Johnson
Metropolitan State College

Ronald F. Kirby
Southeast Missouri State University

Franklin A. Lindeberg
University of California, Riverside

E. Dawn McDonald
Iowa State University

Joan Nessler
Penn State University

John M. Pearson
Central Washington University

Judy Sorensen
University of Arizona

Pat Stock
University of California, Santa Barbara

Helen J. Watt
Temple University

Susan Yates
Fresno Community College

The Series Editor for West's Physical Activities Series

The Series Editor for West's Physical Activities Series is Dr. Bob O'Connor, Los Angeles Pierce College. Dr. O'Connor received his B.S. and M.S. degrees in physical education from UCLA and his doctorate from U.S.C. His 30-year teaching experience includes instruction in physical education courses of tennis, weight training, volleyball, badminton, swimming and various team sports, as well as classes in teaching methods. He brings to the Series a wide range of college coaching experience in areas of swimming, tennis, water polo, and football. Internationally, Dr. O'Connor has been an advisor to several Olympic programs in weight training and swimming. He was among the first to popularize strength training for all athletic events. Dr. O'Connor has written extensively in the fields of physical education and health and is a dedicated advocate of physical education TODAY.

Books in West's Physical Activities Series

Aerobics Today by Carole Casten and Peg Jordan
Badminton Today by Tariq Wadood and Karlyne Tan
Dance Today by Lorraine Person and Marian Weiser
Golf Today by J. C. Snead and John Johnson
Racquetball Today by Lynn Adams and Irwin Goldbloom
Swimming and Aquatics Today by Ron Ballatore and William Miller
Tennis Today by Glenn Bassett and William Otta
Volleyball Today by Marv Dunphy and Rod Wilde
Weight Training Today by Robert O'Connor, Jerry Simmons and, J. Patrick O'Shea

CHAPTER 1
Introduction To Badminton

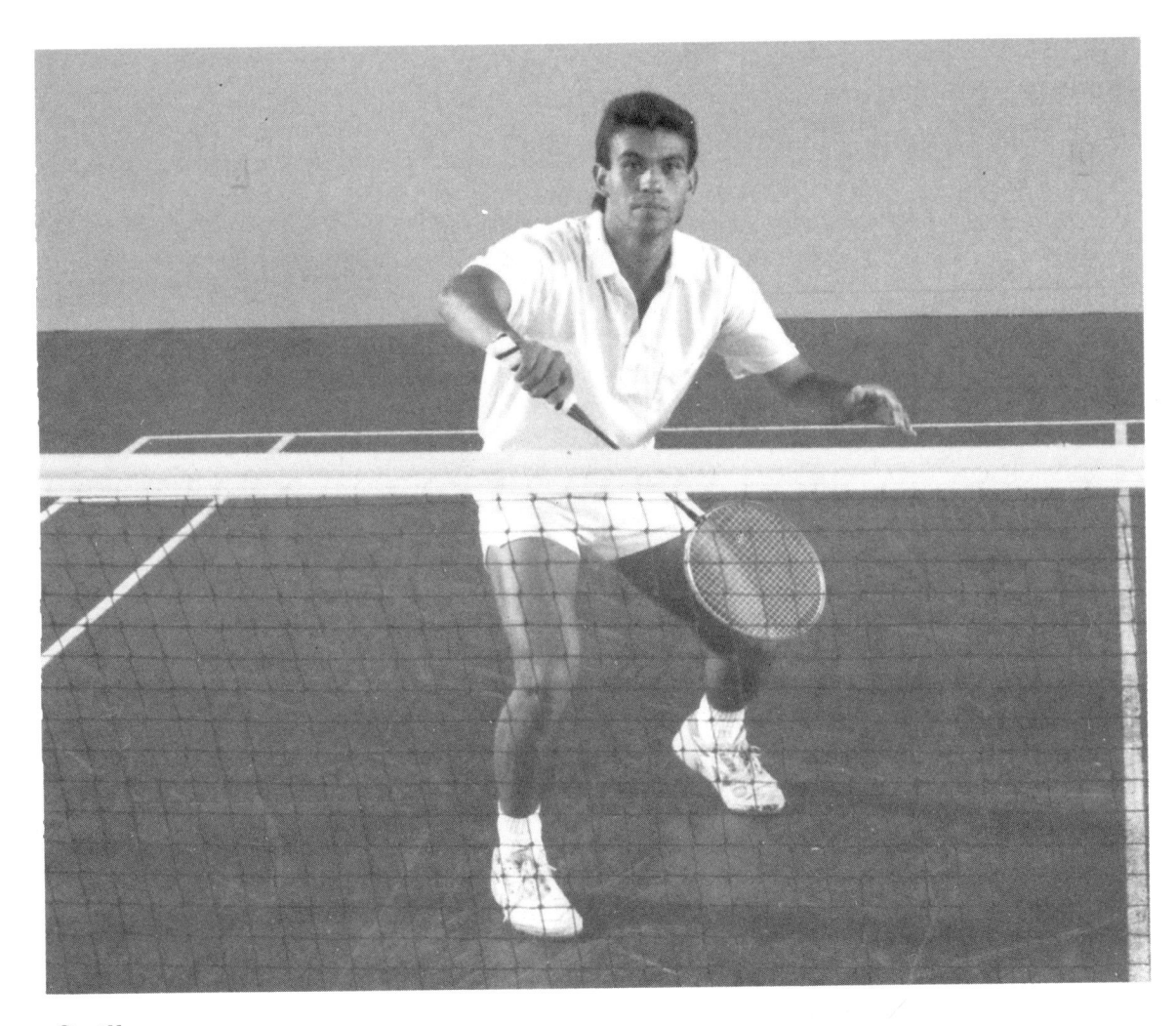

Outline

Benefits of Playing Badminton
History of Badminton
Where to Play Badminton
Checklist on the Basics of the Game
Summary

Badminton is a game in which two players (singles game) or four players (doubles game) hit a light, feathered object (shuttlecock) over a net with their rackets. The objective is to win the game of 15 points (11 points for ladies singles) by hitting the shuttle into the opponent's court and preventing it from landing within the boundaries of your own court.

The strategy of winning involves using a variety of shots to force your opponent to lose the rally. The players attempt to move their opponents around the court, forcing weak returns, or they hit hard shots (smashes) that the opponents cannot return.

Benefits of Playing Badminton

A major benefit of badminton is that it is so easy to learn that it is fun almost as soon as you pick up your racket for the first time. Yet, as your skill level increases, the game involves much more strategy and demands greater physical conditioning. Therefore, your enjoyment of the game should increase as your skill level develops. For these reasons it is one of the most popular sports internationally. At the advanced level it is the fastest court game in the world.

Badminton is also a very social sport. It produces a congenial atmosphere that encourages easy interaction among people of both sexes in both school and club environments. Since the game can be played indoors or outdoors, and its court is relatively small (20 x 44 feet), badminton can be played almost anywhere. This makes it a fine family recreation.

There are obvious physical benefits to the game. The long rallies aid in the development of cardiovascular fitness. The stretching and twisting also aid in developing flexibility. The nature of the game develops an increased level of agility and coordination.

On a psychological level badminton helps reduce tensions as players move around the court and strike the shuttle. Additionally, as they improve in skill, they develop a higher level of self-satisfaction that comes with the accomplishment of any goal.

Badminton, as we know it today, is second only to soccer as the world's most popular participation activity. An activity for all ages and for both sexes, it is a unique and exciting competitive sport. When the shuttle is hit by a skilled player, it can reach a speed well over 200 miles per hour or float delicately over the net. No other sport has as great a variation of speed.

Because of the limited exposure badminton receives in the United States, many people hold the erroneous belief that it is not a vigorous and challenging activity. When observing beginners hitting the shuttle slowly over the net, it becomes easy to draw this conclusion. But given the proper instruction, the players can learn to control the tempo of the game, and it becomes fascinating to watch as well as to play. As the players learn more strokes, the rallies become more exciting.

Many racket sports are difficult and frustrating to learn. In badminton, even beginning players can start a rally almost immediately and gain a sense of achievement. Whether you are playing just for the exercise or planning to enter competition, it is an excellent cardiovascular activity. It requires fast reflexes, good physical conditioning, and concentration.

Furthermore, badminton is a "lifetime sport," not just one for the young.

History of Badminton

While there is some evidence that a game similar to badminton (called *battledore*) was played in China 2,000 years ago, badminton as it is presently played originated in England. The English royal court records refer to a similar sport as early as the twelfth century. Most historians believe that English officers brought the game they called *Poona* to India in the seventeenth century. They then brought it back home again to England in the late nineteenth century. In 1873 they played Poona at the Duke of Beaufort's estate, called Badminton House, near the village of Badminton in Gloucestershire, England. The name of the Duke's estate soon became the name of the game. It was from this time that the game began to develop rapidly as a popular pastime.

The first badminton club was formed in Bath, England, in 1873. The game was introduced to North America in the 1890s. In 1895 the National Badminton Association of America was formed, and in 1899 the first All England championship tournament for men was played. The next year the championship for women was inaugurated.

As the sport gained in popularity, it became necessary to establish the rules, equipment, and court dimensions. Eventually, in 1893 the English Badminton Association was organized to bring some uniformity in competition. The rules, called laws, have changed little since this time period.

In 1909, the shuttle that we use today was introduced. Prior to this time very fast and unpredictable *missiles* made with poultry feathers arbitrarily stuck into a piece of cork were used. The court was originally shaped like a wasp or hourglass. Today the court is rectangular, and the tournament shuttles are made of very uniform goose feathers inserted into a precisely shaped cork base. In earlier days, the racket was heavy, but modern technology has produced a dramatic change in weight.

Since 1929 badminton has increased in popularity in the United States. The game is played in clubs and in competition between high schools and colleges across the country. It will become a full Olympic medal sport starting in 1992. Some colleges are giving athletic scholarships for badminton because it will soon be a National Collegiate Athletic Association (NCAA) sport.

There are many local and national tournaments and a world championship for individuals. In addition, national teams compete for the Thomas Cup (similar to the Davis Cup in tennis) for men and the Uber Cup for women. Three singles matches and two doubles matches decide the winner in each competition.

Where to Play Badminton

Many high schools and colleges have badminton classes and recreation opportunities. Public parks and recreation centers also often offer opportunities to play, as do many YMCAs and YWCAs. Private badminton clubs are located in most parts of the country (see Appendix D). For more specific information contact United States Badminton Association, 501 West Sixth St., Papillion, Nebraska 68046 (phone 402-592-7309).

Checklist on the Basics of the Game

1. Most games are completed with 15 points. All official ladies games end at 11 points.
2. Only the server can score.
3. During a rally the players attempt to get their opponents to miss a shot by forcing them out of position or hitting a hard shot that cannot be returned.

Summary

1. Badminton as we know it originated in England.
2. It is a sport that can be enjoyed at any age—a "lifetime sport."
3. Badminton can be as slow and relaxing or as vigorous and taxing as you want it to be.
4. The game requires speed, finesse, cardiovascular endurance, and strength.

CHAPTER 2

Equipment and Facilities

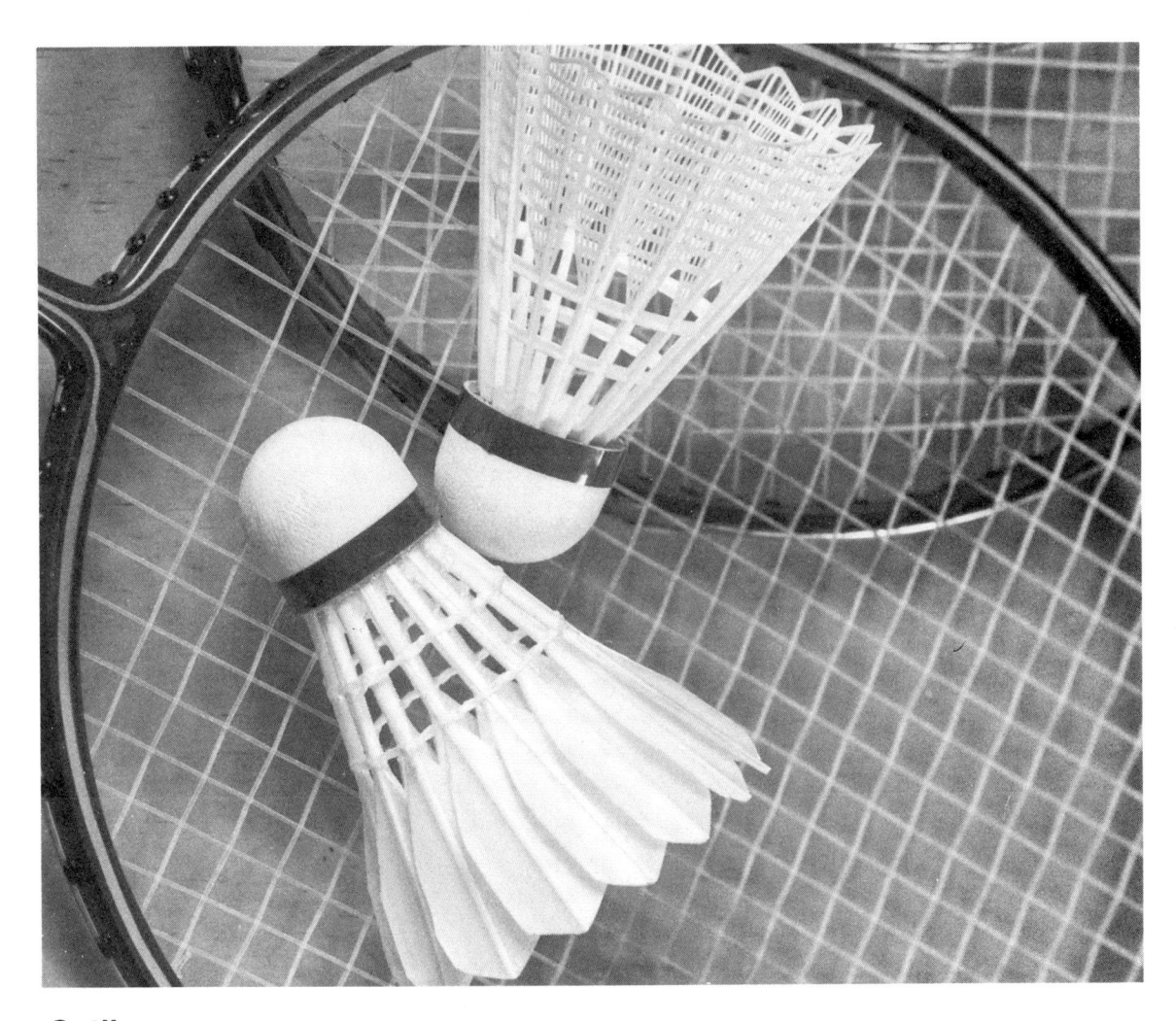

Outline

The Racket
The Shuttle Cock
Clothing
Shoes
Socks

Sweatbands
The Court
Checklist for Game or Practice Equipment
Summary

The Racket

The racket is very light so that it can be moved quickly with a flick of the wrist. It may be made of wood, metal, or synthetic material such as graphite, boron, carbon or ceramic. Beginners do not need an expensive racket, but advanced players may look for special features and special weights that may bring the cost from $40 to $150.

The metal and synthetic rackets are generally stronger and lighter. Because of their strength, they do not need to be placed in a press to retain their shape as the wood rackets require. They can also be strung tighter (17 to 22 pounds) so that the shuttle will fly farther when hit.

The type of game one plays determines the type of racket one should choose. If you enter into competitive badminton you will soon decide whether to be primarily an offensive or a defensive player. An offensive player hits hard and tries to score points that way. A defensive player tries to return every shot back and force the opponent into making mistakes. Every player must have both offensive and defensive skills, but most advanced players will emphasize one style or the other.

Rackets

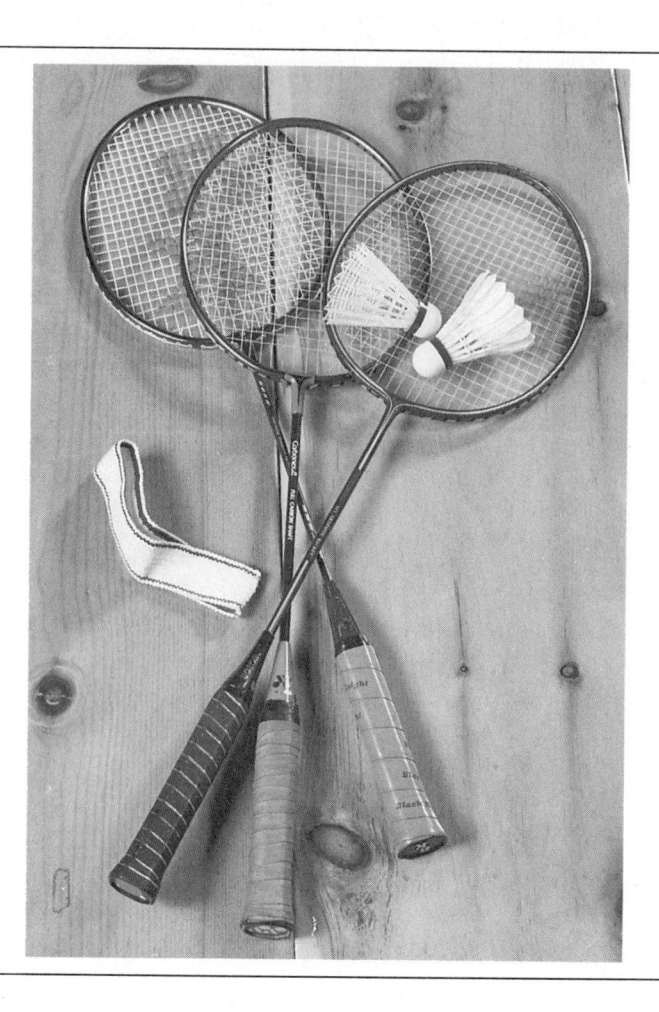

Offensive-minded players generally use rackets more heavily weighted in the head. This gives the player more potential power in a shot. Defensive players use light-headed rackets.

The head, or *face*, of the racket is strung with strings of gut, nylon, or a similar material. Nylon string usually costs less and lasts longer. Tournament players usually use gut, however, because it can be strung with more tension so that the shuttle will bounce from it with more speed.

The *grip* is the part of the handle that is covered with leather or composition. Most companies make only two sizes of grip. Some make three. (The range in circumference is from $3\frac{1}{4}$ to $3\frac{5}{8}$ inches.) The grip should be sufficiently large so that your hand comfortably wraps around it and you feel that it is in no danger of slipping as you hit the shuttlecock.

The Shuttlecock

The *shuttlecock*, usually called the *shuttle* or *bird*, weighs about one-sixth of an ounce (more technically about 4 grams or 73 to 85 grains). The official shuttles are made of goose feathers placed in a cork head that is leather-covered. This is the type of shuttle used in all high-level play. Beginners and school classes often use a cheaper and more durable plastic or nylon shuttle.

Shuttles: feather and plastic

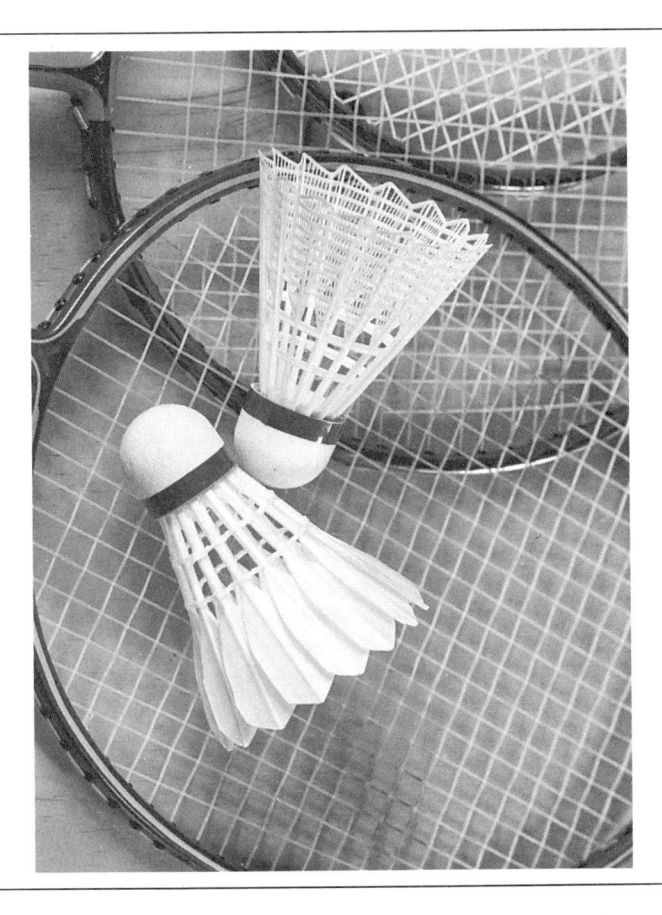

When the temperature is high or you are playing at a higher altitude, the air is thinner. You will then want a lighter shuttle so that it will fall more slowly. Heavier shuttles are used closer to sea level, in climates with a higher humidity, and for outdoor playing.

Clothing

Shorts and shirts are generally worn by both men and women, although some women wear tennis dresses or skirts. The preferred color is white. It helps disguise the white shuttlecock (seen against the backdrop of white clothing)—especially when a player is serving. While most clubs and tournaments allow the same kinds of clothing worn for tennis, some specify a particular type and color. It is wise to check with the director to determine local requirements.

Shirts are generally made of cotton because it has better perspiration-absorption qualities than synthetic fabrics. All clothing should allow you to stretch comfortably.

Shoes

Because of the quick starting and stopping involved in badminton, a tennis shoe is preferred. It should have a non-marking sole with nonskid tread. The preferred color of the shoe is white. Do not use jogging shoes, aerobic shoes, or shoes designed for other sports. They will not give you the lateral foot stability that you need for badminton.

Your shoes should be laced from the bottom eyelets. Pull the laces firm at each higher eyelet. This helps to give you a snug fit and prevent the rubbing that can result in blisters.

Socks

The socks should be wool or cotton to absorb perspiration. In order to avoid blisters you may want to wear two pairs of lighter socks. The two socks rub against each other and reduce the friction between the shoe and the skin that might otherwise result in a blister. The socks should be white.

Sweatbands

If you perspire heavily, you might want to wear a sweatband on your forehead. The sweatband not only reduces the perspiration that can run into your eyes, but it also keeps your hair away from your face. Wristbands prevent perspiration from rolling down your arm and getting your hand sweaty, possibly causing your grip to slip.

The Court

The badminton court is 44 feet long. The singles court is 17 feet wide, while the doubles court is 20 feet wide. The lines are inbounds. The top of the net is 5 feet, 1 inch, at the post and 5 feet at the center of the court.

There is a short service line 6 feet, 6 inches, from the net. The server must stand behind this line, in the service court area, and the serve must clear the opposite short service line to be in play.

EQUIPMENT AND FACILITIES 9

Court: Top view

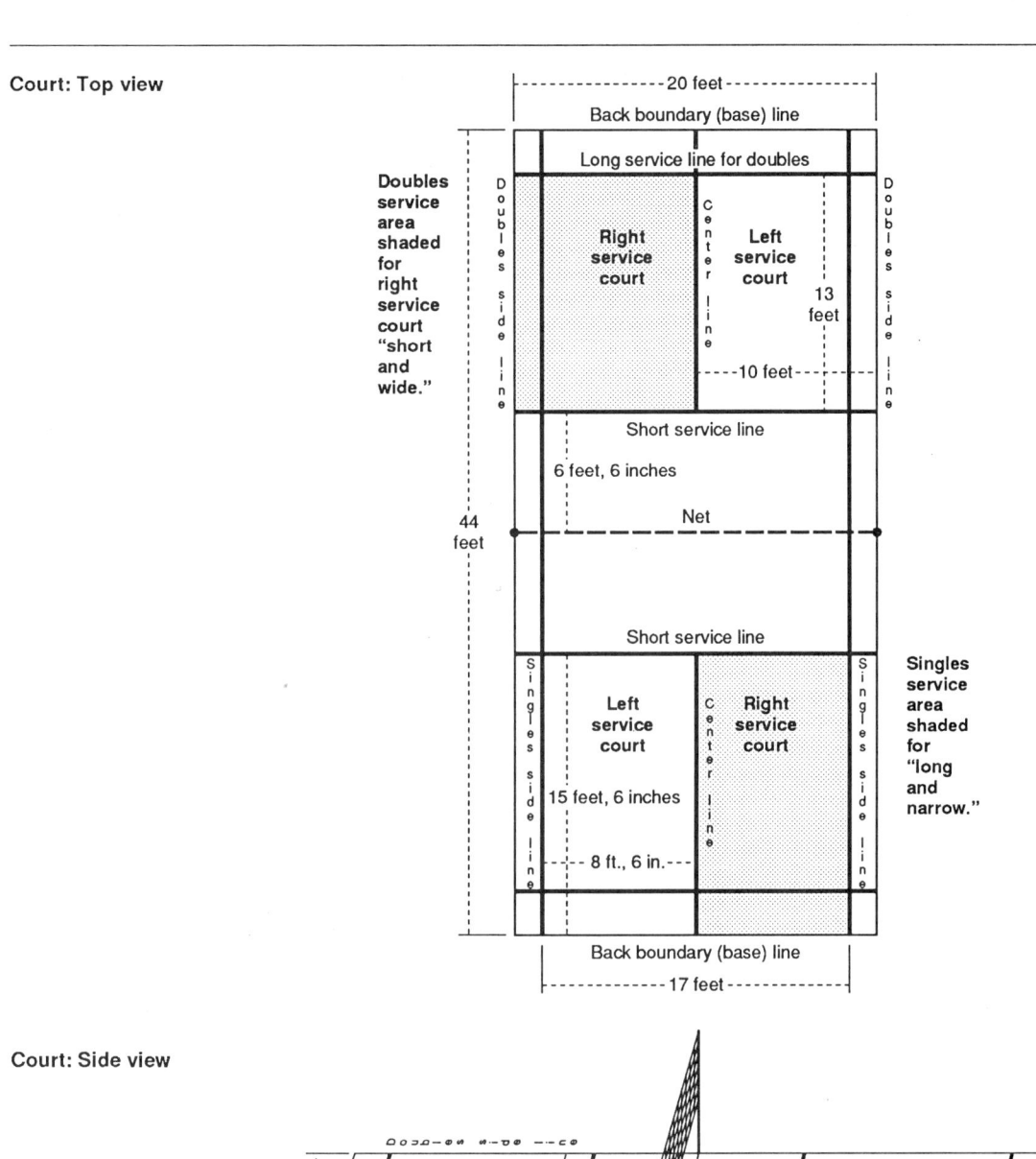

Doubles service area shaded for right service court "short and wide."

- 20 feet
- Back boundary (base) line
- Long service line for doubles
- Doubles side line
- Right service court
- Center line
- Left service court
- 13 feet
- 10 feet
- Short service line
- 6 feet, 6 inches
- Net
- 44 feet
- Short service line
- Singles side line
- Left service court
- Center line
- Right service court
- 15 feet, 6 inches
- 8 ft., 6 in.
- Back boundary (base) line
- 17 feet

Singles service area shaded for "long and narrow."

Court: Side view

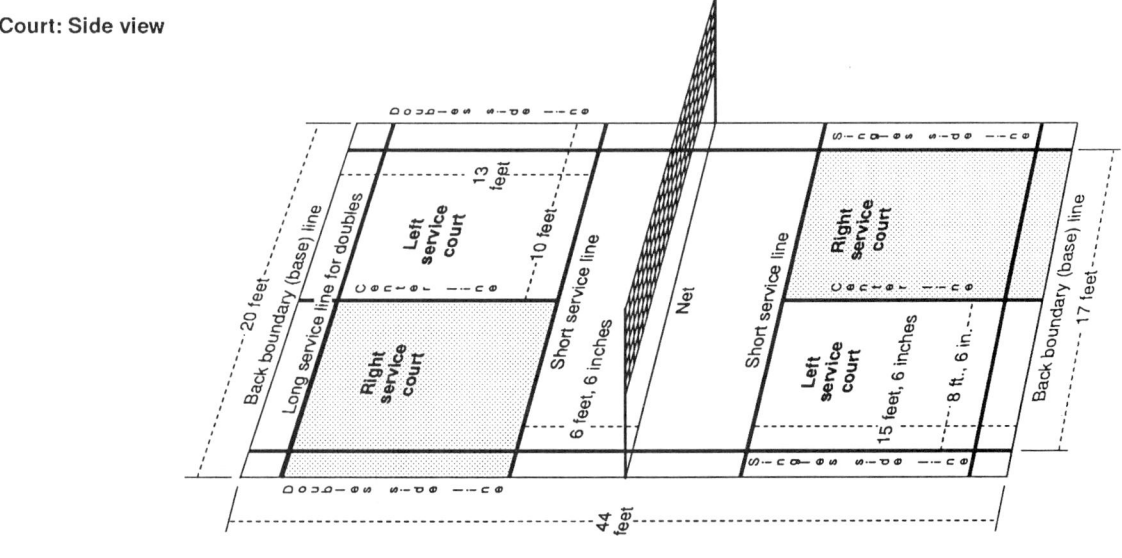

Checklist for Game or Practice Equipment

1. One or two rackets.
2. Two tubes of shuttlecocks.
3. Shoes and socks.
4. Towel.
5. Sweatbands for forehead and wrist (optional).
6. Shirt and shorts.

The serving court for singles is bounded by the short service line, the centerline, the singles sideline, and the back boundary of the court. This produces a long, narrow court 15 feet, 6 inches, long and 8 feet, 6 inches, wide. The server must stand within this court and serve into the diagonally opposite singles court in order to have a legal serve.

The doubles service court is shorter but wider than the singles court. It is bounded by the short service line in front, the centerline, the doubles sideline, and a line 2 feet, 6 inches, in from the rear boundary. The doubles server must stand in this court and serve to the diagonally opposite doubles court to begin play.

There should be at least 20 feet of clearance overhead—24 to 30 feet is considered ideal. A 30-foot ceiling is required for national and international competition.

Summary

1. Rackets can be made of wood, metal, or other materials.
2. Offensive players generally use a racket heavier in the head than the racket defensive players would choose.
3. The shuttlecock can be made of feathers and cork or plastic. The plastic or nylon shuttle plays longer, but the feathers give a better flight and a steeper drop.
4. Clothing should be comfortable enough to allow you to run unimpaired and to stretch easily. The preferred color is white.
5. Shoes should be tennis or all-court shoes with a good nonskid sole.

CHAPTER 3

Laws and Courtesies of the Game

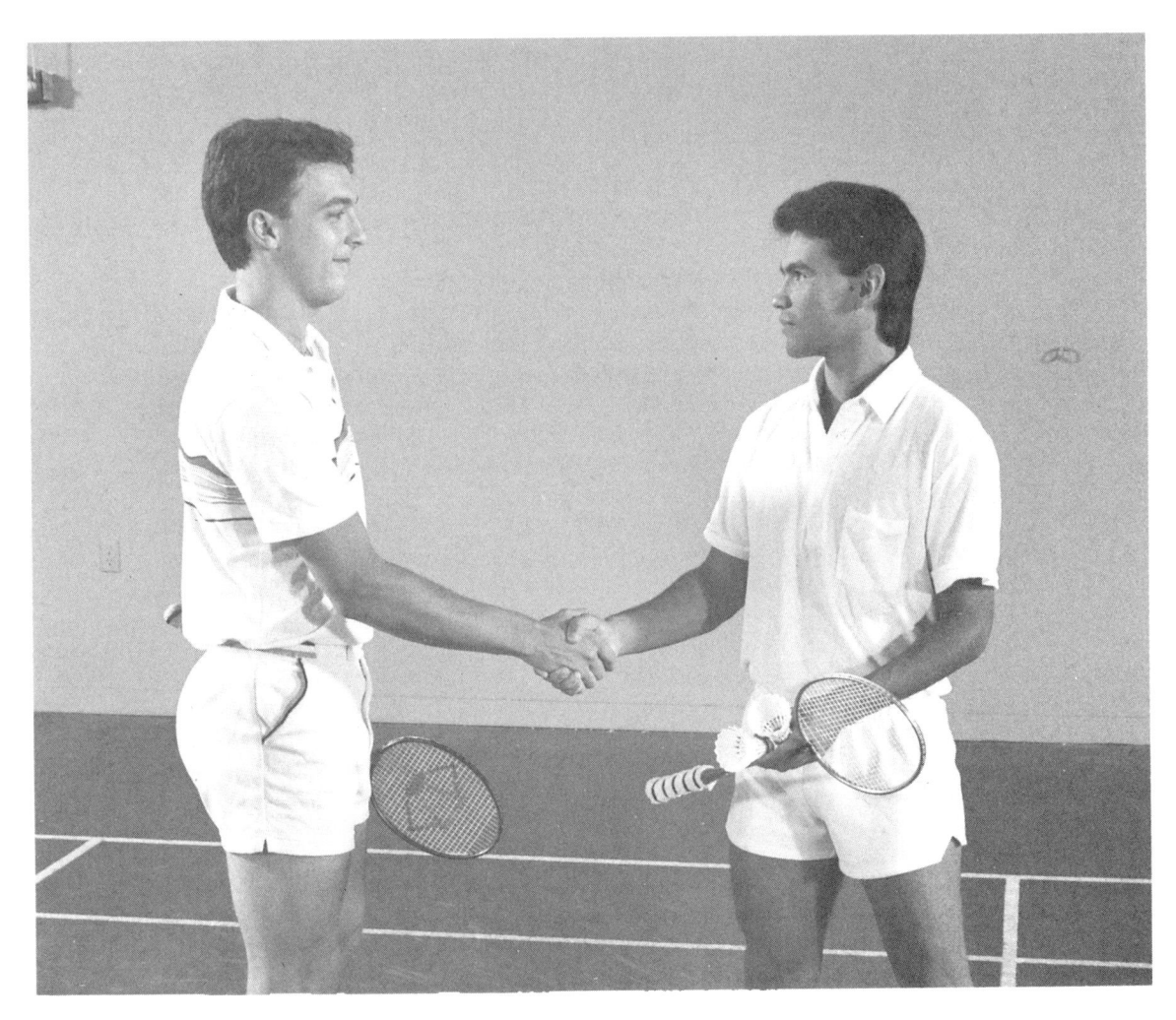

Outline

Courtesies
Simplified Laws (Rules) of Badminton
Checklist for Serving Faults
Summary

Courtesies

The game of badminton emphasizes good sportsmanship, expressed through certain playing *courtesies*. It is expected that you will be friendly to and respectful of your opponent, and gracious whether winning or losing. In addition, here are some specific courtesies expected from those who play badminton.

1. Introduce yourself to your partner and to your opponents before the match. Be sure to shake hands after the match.
2. While warming up, help your opponent's warm-up as well; don't kill every stroke.
3. If there is any question on whether or not you have fouled, call it on yourself.
4. When you are in doubt about whether a shuttle landed in or out, always give the benefit of the doubt to your opponent or replay the point.
5. Never question your opponent's calls.
6. While there are times during a match in which you may want to aim a smash at your opponent, do not do it if you can get the point any other way. If you have a set-up, hit it somewhere else in the court.
7. Control your anger. Never throw your racket.

Opponents shaking hands

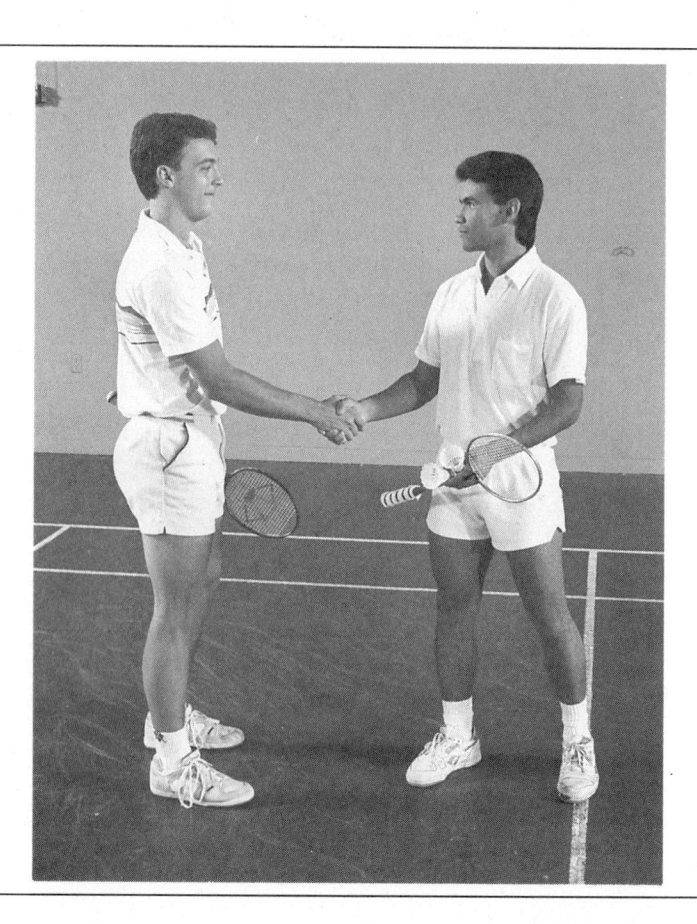

8. Never deride or make fun of an opponent.
9. As the server, keep the score and call it before each serve—calling the server's score first.
10. When your opponent is serving and a shuttle lands on your side of the court, pick it up and hit it back, or toss it under the net to the server.
11. Compliment your opponent on any good shots made.
12. Do not offer advice or criticism to your partner or your opponents.
13. Bring your share of shuttlecocks to every practice and game.
14. Keep up the play. Do not stall between points.
15. Do not talk to your partner during a rally except when you are directing tactics, as in, "I've got it," or "You're up."
16. If you are receiving, be ready to return the shuttle as soon as the server is ready to serve.

Simplified Laws (Rules) of Badminton

The complete laws of the game will be found in Appendix A of this book. A summary follows:

1. Toss for the serve. You can flip a coin, spin a racket, or toss a shuttle to determine who gets the choice of "side or serve." If spinning a racket, identify a marking on the racket then spin it in the hand or on the floor. One person calls the mark. If it is called correctly that person gets the choice. The most common method of determining the choice, however, is by hitting or tossing the shuttle into the air and letting it land. The person towards whom the base of the shuttle is pointing gets the choice. If the winner of the toss

Deciding who serves first by a toss of the shuttle

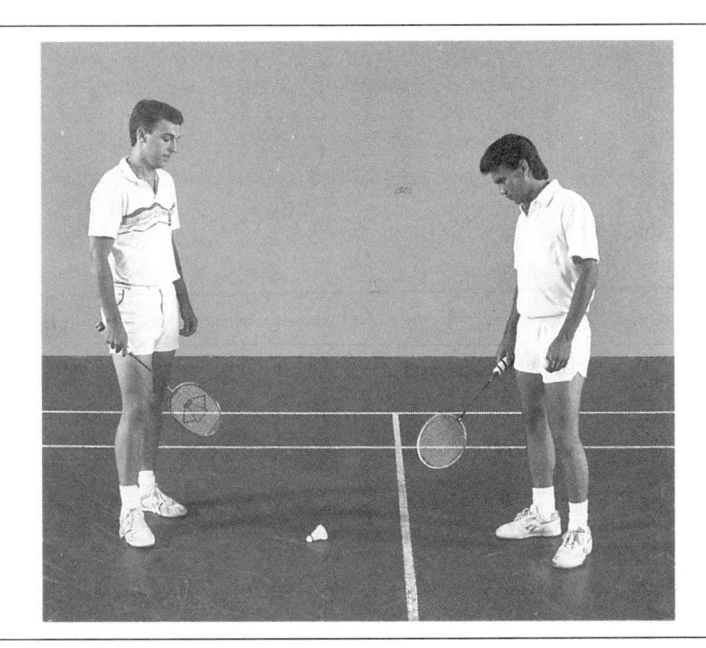

chooses a side of the court to defend, the other person can choose to serve or receive.

The side of the court may become important if one side has poorer lighting or an undesirable background. In an important match the player who wins the toss might elect to defend the less desirable side first. This would then have him or her on the best side for the last half of the third game.

2. Men's games and doubles are played to 15 points but official women's singles play is 11 points.

In a 15-point game, if the score is tied at 13–13, the player who scored 13 first can decide to play two more points and finish the game at 15 (called *no set*) or play five more points to finish the game. If the latter is chosen, the score is started at zero and played to 5 points. If the game is tied at 14–14, the player who scored 14 first can choose to play one more point (no set) or three more points. Once the score is set, the player who tied the score continues to serve. If the player who reached the tied score first does not call to set the score before the server serves, the option to set the score is lost.

In an 11-point game, if the game is tied at 9–9, the first person to score 9 points has the option of playing two points (no set) or three more points. If the game is tied at 10, the choice would be between one (no set) or two more points.

3. The serve, if not played by the receiver, must land in the diagonal service court. Any shuttle hitting the line is *in*. In singles the shuttle must land in the long, narrow court. In doubles it must land in the short, wide court. In doubles the long service line is for the service boundary only. Once the serve has been hit, the full court (20 x 44 feet) is played.

In singles the serve is made from the right service court whenever the server's score is an even number (0, 2, 4, etc.). The serve is from the left court whenever the server's score is an odd number (1, 3, 5, etc.)

In doubles the serve is always started from the right court. The first server in doubles will serve from the right court. If the point is won, the server will serve next from the left court. The server will alternate sides until the serve is lost. The players on both teams should remember where they were during the first service, because they will have to be in those same positions whenever the server's score is even. The returners will always defend the same service court during an *inning*, that is, the time that a player or team holds service. (Once the serve has been returned, the players can move anyplace in the court.) The servers will change courts whenever they score.

In doubles the first server serves until the serving team commits a fault, and the serve is lost. This is called *one hand down*. When the first serving team loses the serve, the opponent in the right court (the receiver in the first hand) will serve and will continue to serve until the serve is lost. Then the server's partner will serve until the serve

Correct serve

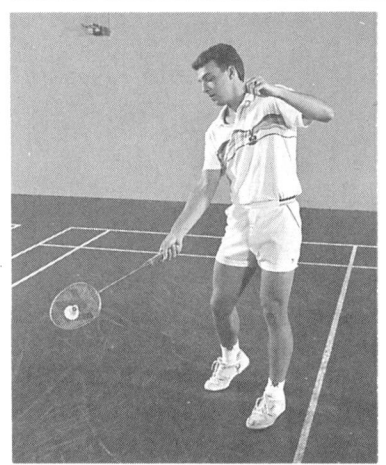

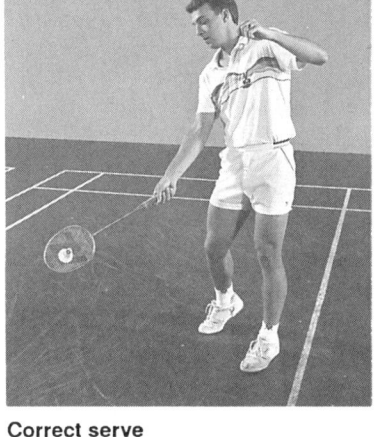

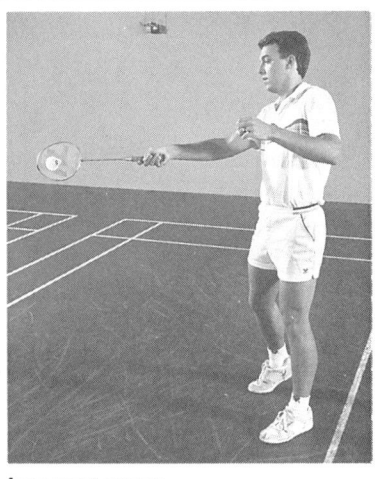

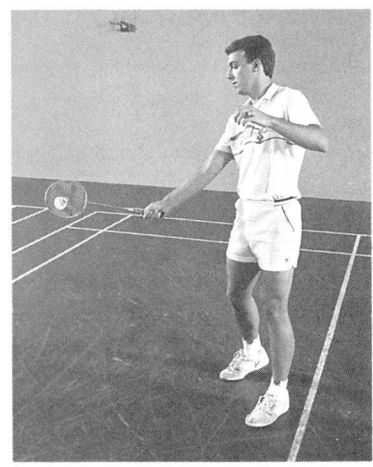

Incorrect serve:
A. Above the waist

B. Racket head above the hand

is lost—*two hands down*. The players on the team which began serving in the match will then each get a turn and serve until losing.

4. The server has only one chance to serve the shuttle over the net and into the proper court. The shuttle may hit the net and land in the proper court and be legal.
5. Most matches are "best two out of three games." The winner of the match will be the one who wins two games. The players will change sides of the court after each game. If a third game is required, the players will switch ends after 8 points in a 15-point game and after 6 points in an 11-point game.
6. *Faults* (loss of serve for the serving team or loss of the point for the receiving team) occur whenever
    a. A serve is illegal for the following reasons:
       1. The shuttle is hit when it is above the waist.
       2. The head of the racket is above the hand when the shuttle is hit.
       3. The server misses the shuttle when trying to hit it.
    b. Any serve or other shot does one of the following:
       1. Goes under or through the net.
       2. Hits an overhead obstruction.
       3. Hits a player inside or outside of the court.
    c. A serve lands outside the proper service area.
    d. A shot lands out of bounds (only if the head, not the feathers of the shuttle lands outside the lines).
    e. Either the server or receiver steps out of the proper court before the shuttle is served.
    f. The receiving player does not play the shuttle. (Only the proper receiver may return the serve.)

Reaching over the net to return the shuttle

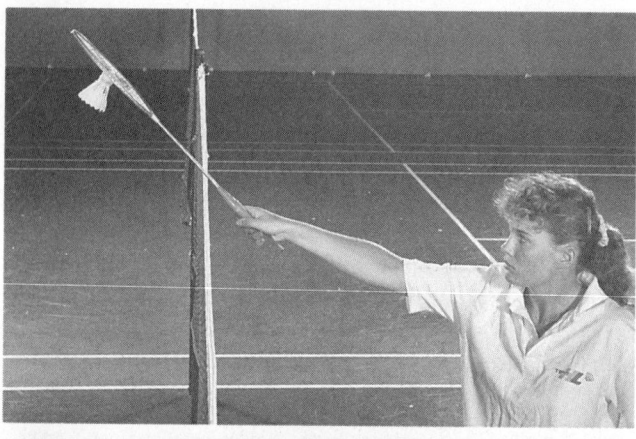

Touching the net with the racket

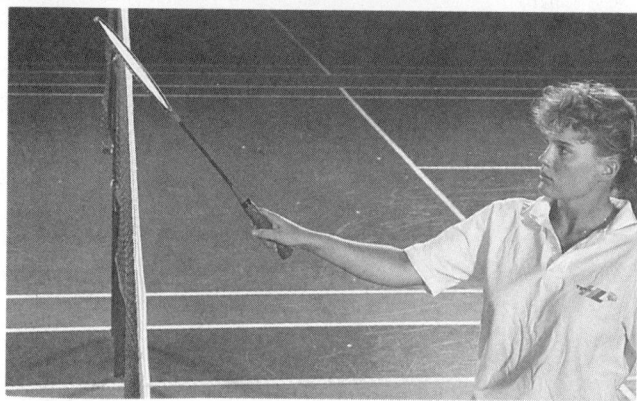

g. A player reaches over the net to hit the shuttle. (It is legal to follow through over the net provided that the player or racket does not hit the net.)

h. A player touches the net with the racket or any part of the body or clothing.

Checklist for Serving Faults

1. When serving, the shuttle must be hit with the entire racket head below the waist.
2. The head of the racket must be below the hand when the shuttle is hit.
3. The shuttle must not hit anyone before the receiver has the opportunity of hitting it. (The shuttle may hit the net.)
4. The server must have both feet in contact with the floor when beginning the serve.

i. A player hits the shuttle twice (a *double hit*) or carries it on the racket (rather than having it bounce quickly from the strings) before it crosses the net.
j. The server steps forward when serving.
k. A player obstructs or hinders an opponent.
l. A player catches the shuttle and calls it *out*.

Summary

1. Badminton is a game in which good sportsmanship is expected.
2. The courtesies spell out the expected behavior of a badminton player.
3. The laws of badminton allow for 11-point games (for women's singles) and for the 15-point game (for men's singles and all doubles games).
4. When the game is tied at 1 or 2 points away from the expected game-ending score, the player or team who reached that score first may set the score at which the game will end.
5. The shuttle cannot be double-hit.
6. The lines are in.

CHAPTER 4

Grips, Footwork, and the Ready Position

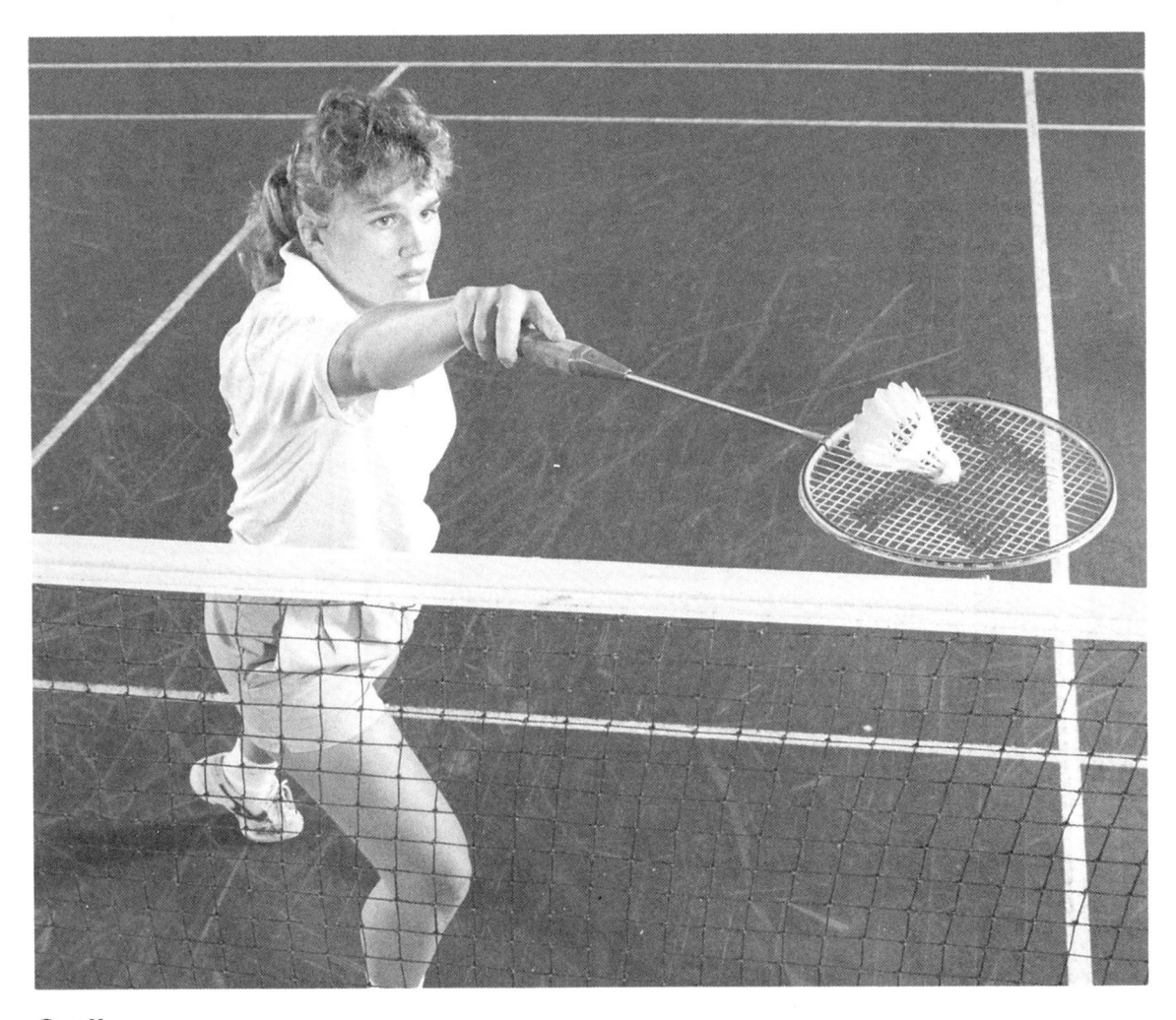

Outline

Grips
 Forehand Grip
 Backhand Grip
 Frying-Pan Grip
Checklist for the Forehand Grip
Checklist for the Backhand Grip
The Ready Position
 Rally Ready
 Ready Position for Return of Service

Home Base for Singles Games
Checklist for Ready Position
Footwork
Warming Up
Checklist for the Warm-Up
Cooling Down
Summary

Grips

The basics of badminton skills start with the grip. Without the proper grip you will not be able to execute strokes effectively or efficiently. There are two essential grips—the forehand and the backhand. The following description is for right-handed players. If you are left-handed just reverse the instructions. Remember that whichever grip you use, you should check it often to make sure it is correct.

Forehand Grip
Hold the head of your racket perpendicular to the floor and "shake hands" with the grip on the handle of the racket. There will be a "V" formed by the juncture of your thumb and index finger. It should be slightly left of center on the top of the grip. The grip should be with your fingers, not the palm of your hand. Your fingers should be slightly spread, with your forefinger extended even farther out. The grip is different from the way you would grip a hammer.

Your thumb wraps around the handle and rests on the side of the middle finger. The palm of the hand should be parallel with the face of the racket. The butt of the racket handle should be touching the heel of your hand.

The grip should be rather loose. A tight grip will cause tension in your hand and wrist and will restrict the wrist action that is so essential to a badminton shot. As you hit a shot, you will tighten your grip somewhat. When you hit a hard shot, you will tighten your grip more than on softer shots.

Backhand Grip
For strokes taken on the backhand (non-racket) side of the body, the grip must be changed to a backhand grip. Otherwise, the racket face will point slightly upward and you will not have control of the shot.

Forehand grip:

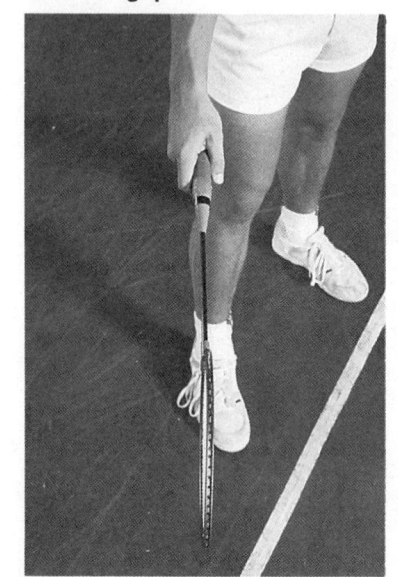

A. From above: right

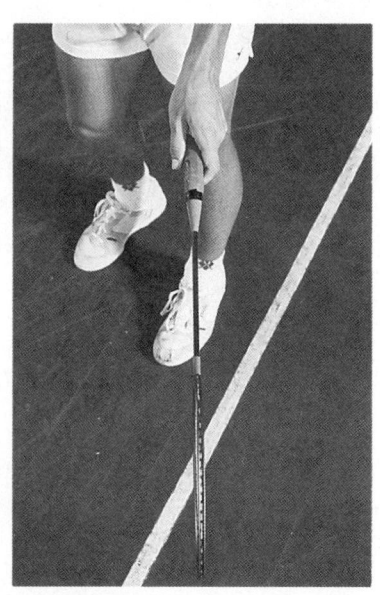

B. From above: left

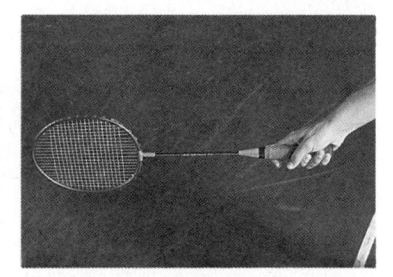

C. From side: right

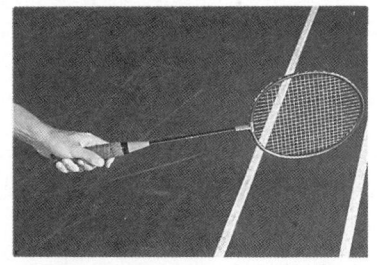

D. From side: left

GRIPS, FOOTWORK, AND THE READY POSITION 21

Forehand grip (cont'd):

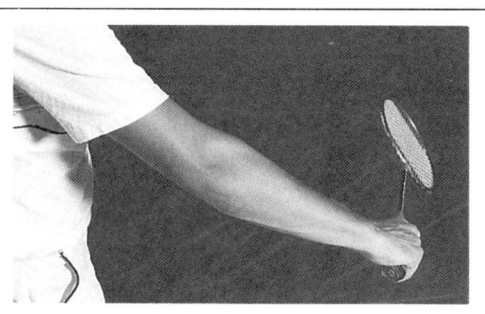

E. From back: right

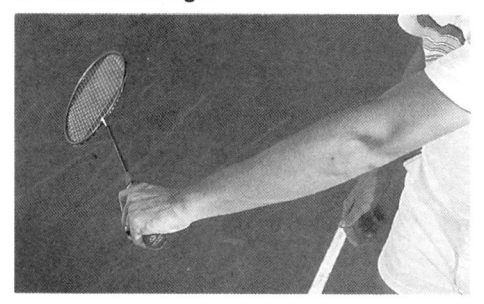

F. From back: left

There are two types of backhand grips. The first has the racket moved a quarter-turn clockwise (so that as your thumb moves farther behind the racket, the back of your hand moves toward the top of the handle). The knuckle of your index finger will now be on the top of the handle, and your thumb will be behind the handle, pointing up the shaft. The "V" formed at the base of your thumb and index finger will now be over the top bevel of the handle.

Backhand grip:

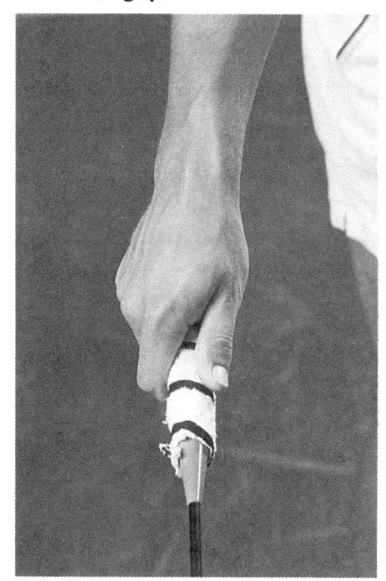

A. From above: right

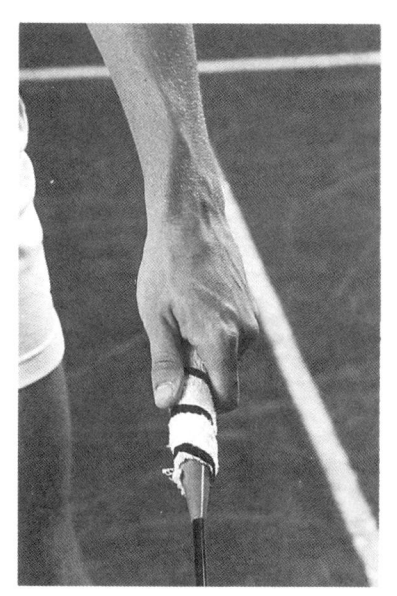

B. From above: left

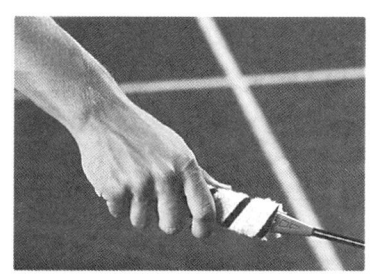

C. From side: right

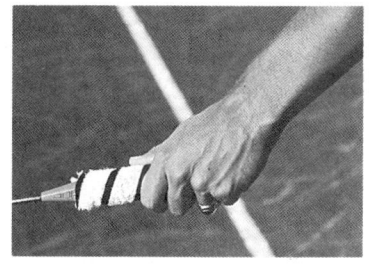

D. From side: left

Backhand grip (cont'd):

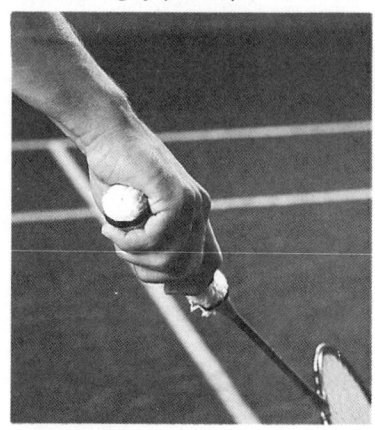

E. From back: right

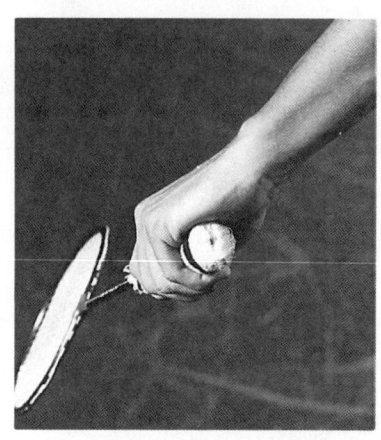

F. From back: left

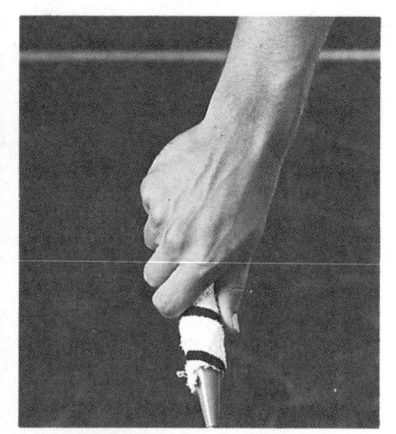

G. Backhand grip changing thumb position

Some players believe that they have more power with this technique. The disadvantage is for shots behind you. In this case the grip loses some of its effectiveness. This is also the grip used in the backhand serve.

The second type of backhand grip changes only the position of the thumb from the forehand grip. It moves from behind the handle to a position along the upper left corner of it. This grip is more efficient for shots behind you. Some players prefer it for other shots as well.

Frying-Pan Grip

Sometimes used by more advanced players, the so-called frying-pan grip is used primarily in doubles play at the net and for service returns. To get the feel of this grip, place the racket on the floor and grasp it like a frying pan, about an inch above the end of the handle. This is also known as the western grip.

Frying-pan grip

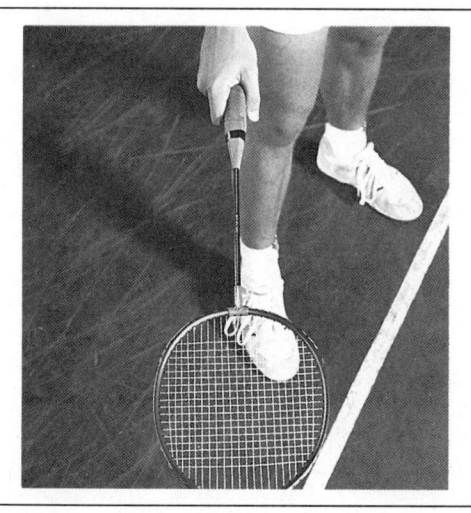

GRIPS, FOOTWORK, AND THE READY POSITION 23

Checklist for the Forehand Grip

1. With the racket head perpendicular to the floor, is the "V" formed by the thumb and index finger on top of the handle grip?
2. Is the index finger separated from the middle finger by resting higher on the handle?
3. Is the grip loose rather than tight?
4. Is the racket held in the fingers rather than in the palm of your hand?

Checklist for the Backhand Grip

1. Did you move your hand a quarter-turn toward the back side of the handle?
2. Is the first knuckle of the index finger on top of the handle?
3. Is your thumb behind the handle and pointing up the shaft?

The Ready Position

Rally Ready

The rally-ready position is taken whenever you are ready to hit a shot, whether it be a smash, a drive, or a drop. From this position you will be best able to move effectively forward or back and right or left. It is similar to the "ready position" for most sports. Your feet should be spread to shoulder width or slightly wider. Your ankles and knees should be slightly flexed, and you should be bent forward at the waist. Your weight should be slightly on the balls of your feet so that you are ready to move in any direction. (If you curl your toes down just a bit, you will feel your weight on the forward part of your feet.)

Your arms should be forward, with the racket-holding hand at about waist height—ready to move to a forehand or backhand hit. And you should be relaxed, because you can move more quickly when you are relaxed than when you are tense.

Ready Position for Return of Service

This position is slightly different. You will keep your non-racket foot (left foot for right-handers) forward. This will allow you to move more quickly up and back as necessary to return a service. The racket head will be in front of your right shoulder for right-handers or the left shoulder for left-handers.

Rally-ready position:

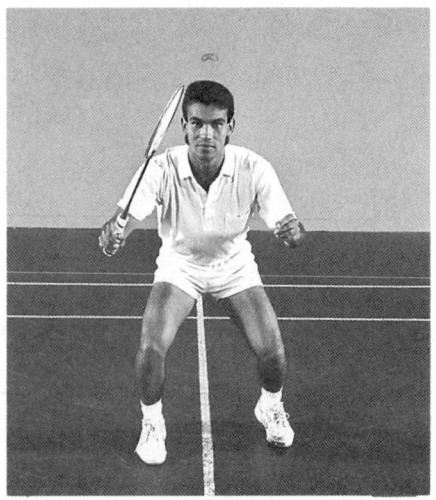

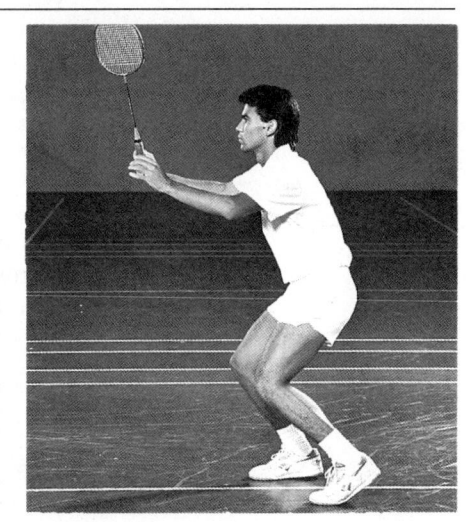

A. From front

B. From side

Ready position for return

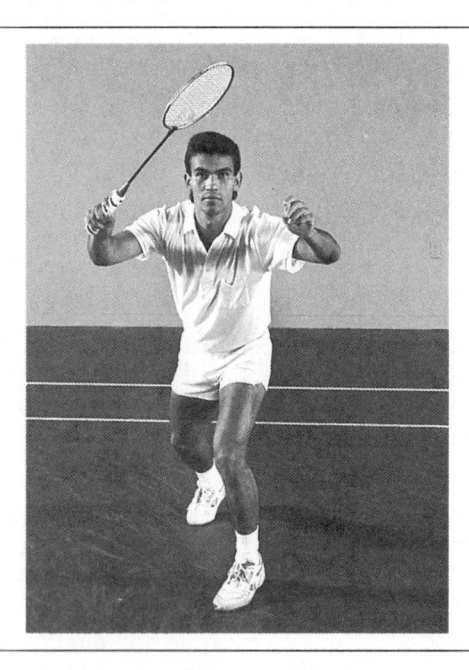

If the serve is behind you, push off your left foot, and run or shuffle back to the spot where you will hit the shuttle. If the serve is hit short, bring your right foot forward and attack the shuttle.

Home Base for Singles Games

In badminton you do not have time to get ready for most shots as you do in tennis or golf. For this reason you must *always* be ready to react to the shuttle. The best position from which to defend your court is in the middle of the court—on the centerline, a few feet ahead of a spot halfway between the net and the

Checklist for the Ready Position

1. Are you in the center of the court?
2. Are your shoulders square to the net?
3. Are your feet spread slightly wider than your shoulders with your weight on the balls of your feet?
4. Are your ankles, knees, and hips slightly flexed so that you are ready to move in any direction?
5. Are you holding the racket with a forehand grip and with the racket forward of the midline of your body?
6. Are you ready to move in any direction quickly?

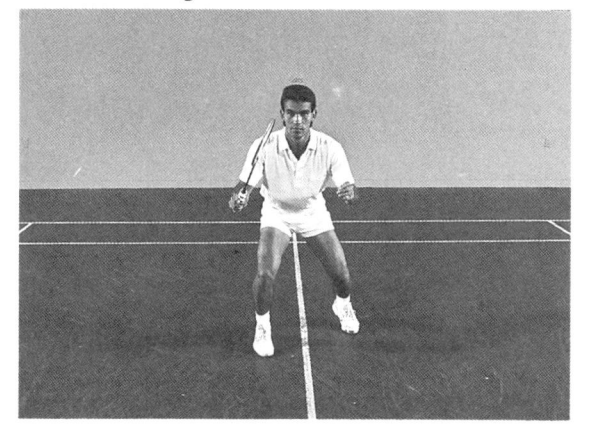

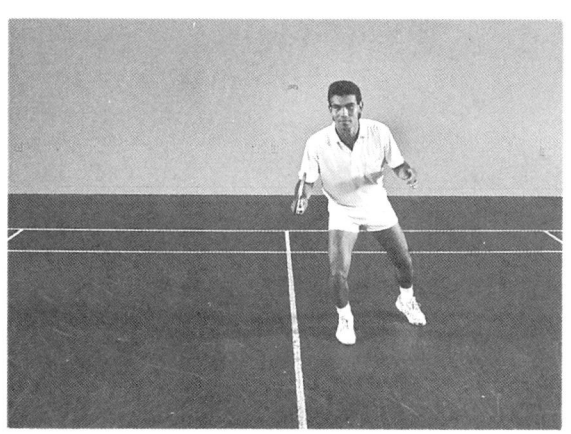

Home base: singles

back boundary line. (This puts you about 2 feet behind the "T" that is formed by the centerline meeting the front service line.) From this position you can get to the front court to handle the drop shots and will still have time to move back to play the clears.

Depending on your individual strength and quickness, you might want to play a few feet ahead or behind this center area. Your home-base position may also vary depending on your opponent. You might play farther forward if the opponent is weaker or uses a lot of drop shots. You might play farther back against a strong smasher or clearing player.

As you become more advanced, you may move a bit to one side or the other to take away your opponent's angle of return. When you hit to a deep corner, your opponent has a greater angle in which to return to your court. If you hit to the center of the court, the angle is reduced.

Always try to get to home base after every shot. However, if your opponent is ready to hit the shuttle and you haven't yet returned to your home base, stop and get set to defend your court from wherever you are on the court.

Center position for shot down middle

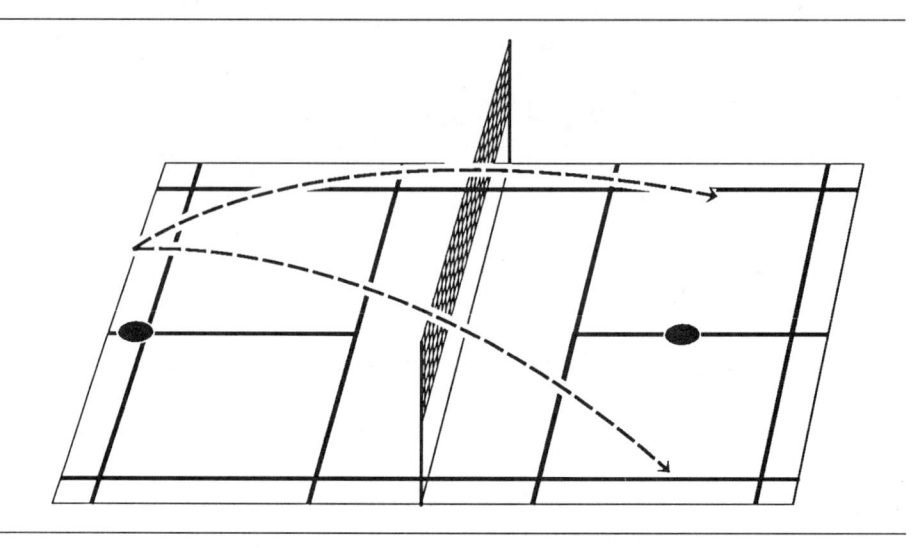

Angle of return:
A. With opponent in deep right corner

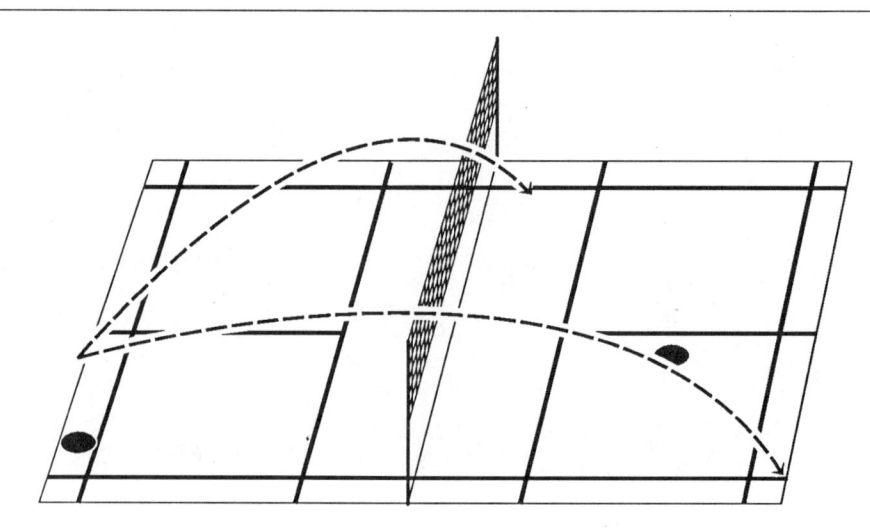

B. With opponent in deep left corner

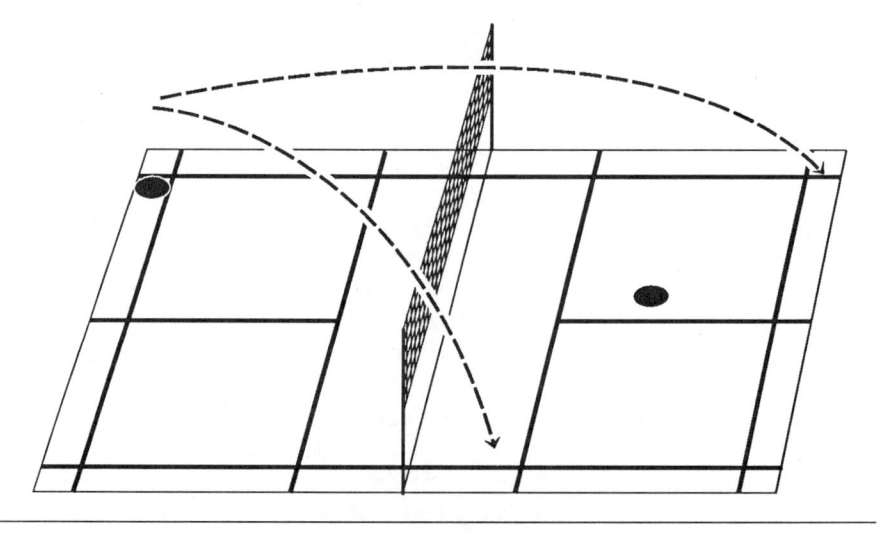

Footwork

Good footwork is essential in badminton. You must be able to get to the shuttle quickly before you can hit your stroke. Being a little slow getting into position will force you to make a less effective shot. For example, not being behind a smash will greatly reduce the downward angle of the shot and may make the shuttle go too high or too long.

Footwork:

A. Push-off on left foot going right

B. Turn sideways on deep shots

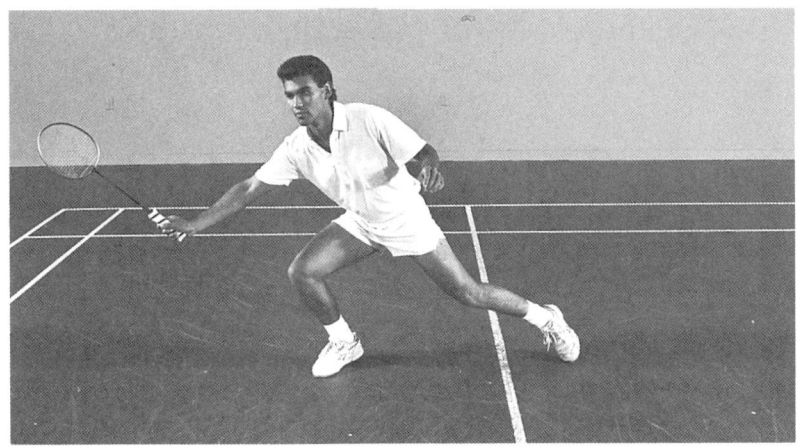

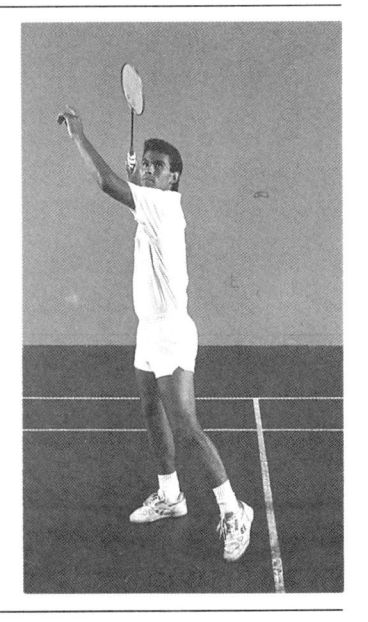

From your ready position you should be able to move quickly as your opponent hits the shuttle. Watch the shuttle as it leaves your opponent's racket, and push off hard with the foot that is away from where you want to move—your left foot if you are moving to the right. Keep your feet low to the ground to avoid wasted motion.

For deep shots get your body turned sideways so that your chest is facing the sideline near the shuttle. For shots close to the net, your final step will be with your racket side foot (right foot for right-handers).

The best way to improve footwork is *shadow practice*. Simply have someone on the other side of the net point to a spot where the imaginary shuttle is flying. Move quickly to that position and swing as if you were hitting the shuttle. Quickly return to the base position, in the center of the court, after each shot.

For shots hit close to the net, remember that you will always hit the shot with your racket-side foot closest to the point of contact. (Right foot for right-handers.) If the shuttle is a long way away, step with the left foot first, then with the right foot. If it is close, just step with the right foot.

For shots deep in the court, the more advanced players will scissor their legs as they hit. The right foot may be back while the backswing is being completed, but the player will jump and hit, switching the legs and gaining ground back toward the base position.

Step with racket foot towards net on shots hit close to the net:

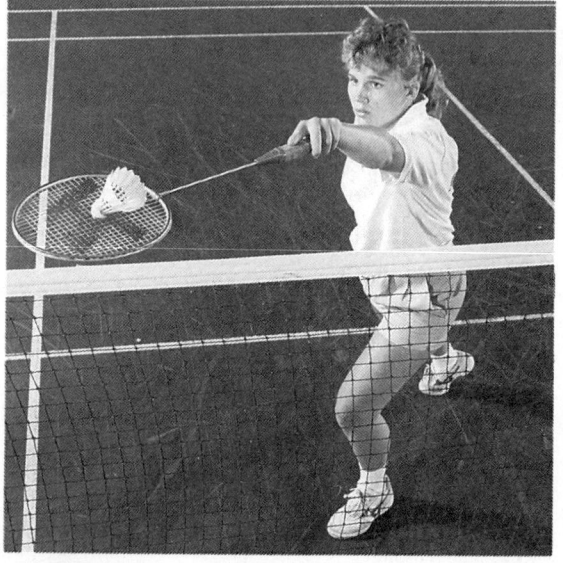

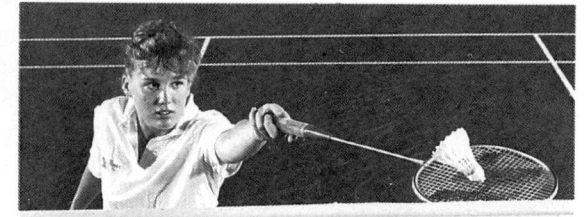

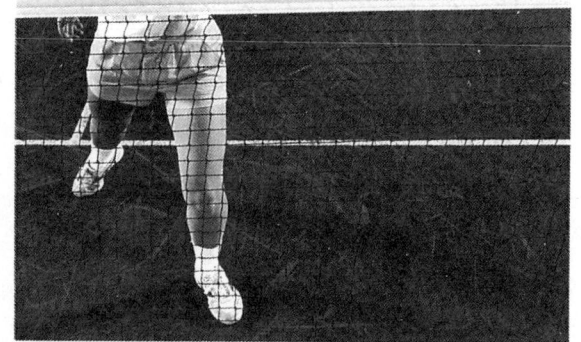

A. Right Court

B. Left Court

Scissors step on smash

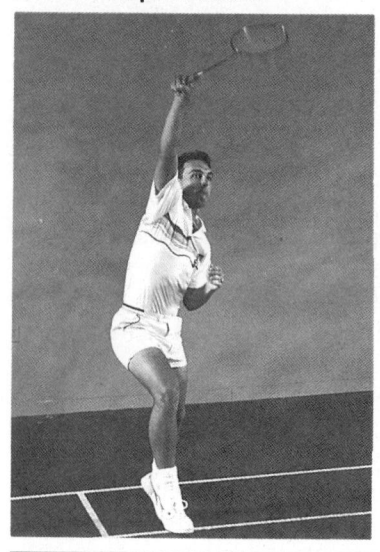

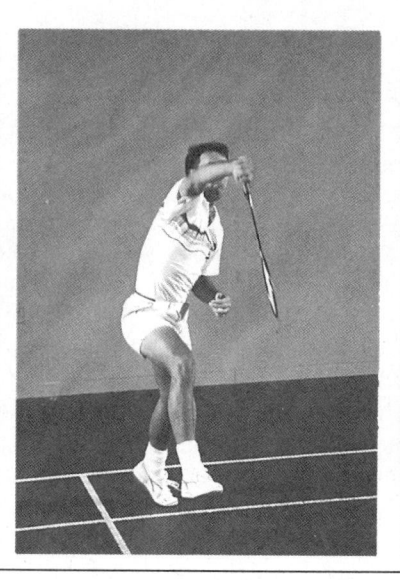

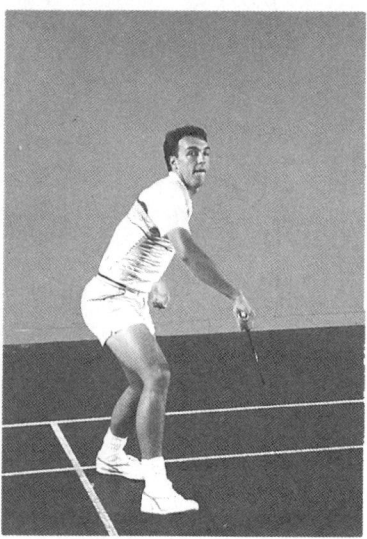

Warming Up

As in any physical sport, badminton players must prepare their bodies for the rigors of the game. The warm-up should include stretching and moving your muscles so that you will be able to move quickly when the game starts. A proper warm-up also helps avoid injuries to muscles and joints during the game. Some guidelines follow:

GRIPS, FOOTWORK, AND THE READY POSITION 29

Arm circles

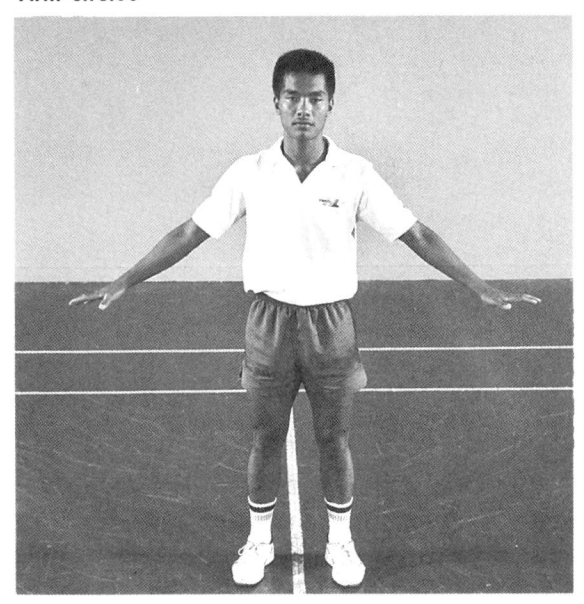

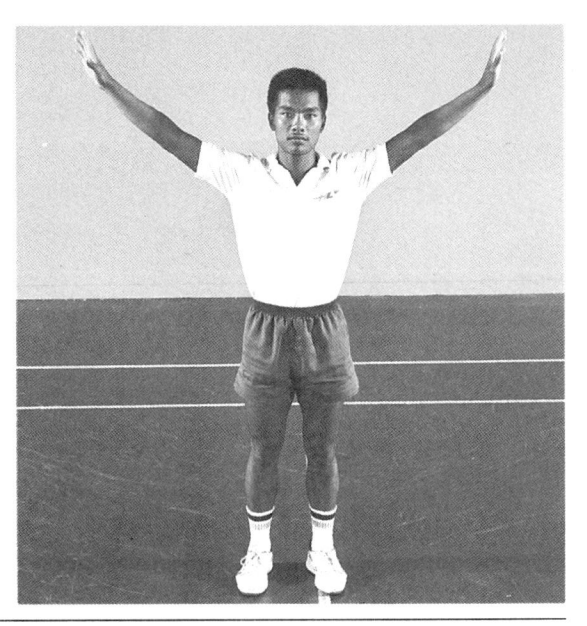

1. Jog around the gym, or do relaxed jumping jacks for a minute. This warms up your muscles and allows your body to stretch more efficiently.
2. Swing your arms in big circles forward and back—ten times each.
3. With your feet spread, reach up high with your right arm, then twist your whole body right for 20 seconds. Next, raise your left arm and twist left for 20 seconds.
4. With one foot 3 to 5 feet ahead of the other, and both feet flat on the floor, step far forward on one foot while allowing the calf muscle of

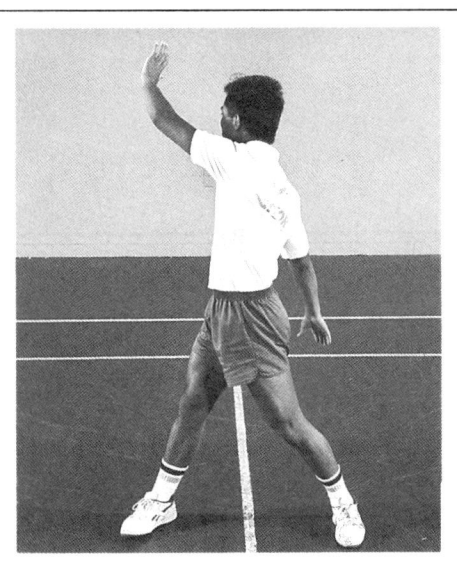

A. Side stretch

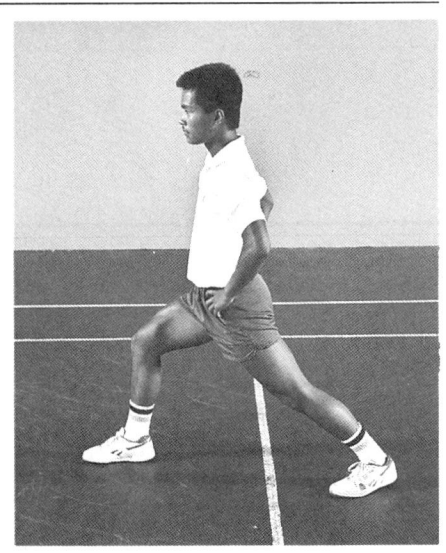

B. Calf stretch

Sitting toe touch

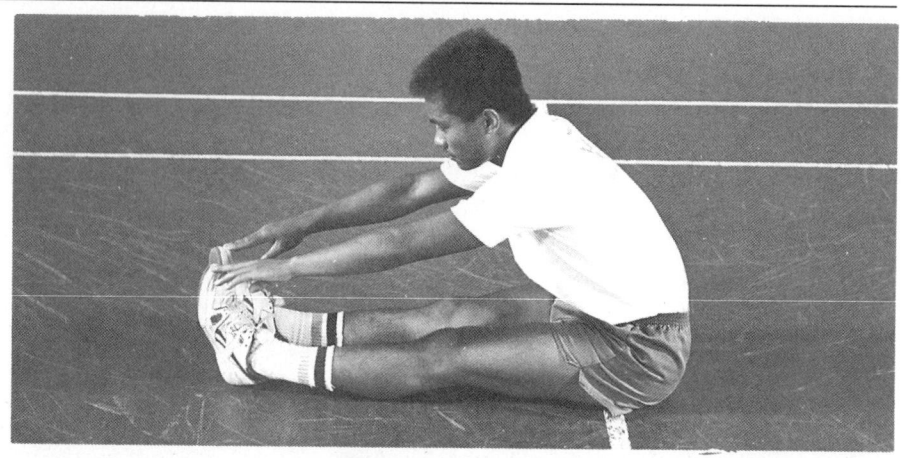

Strattle groin stretch

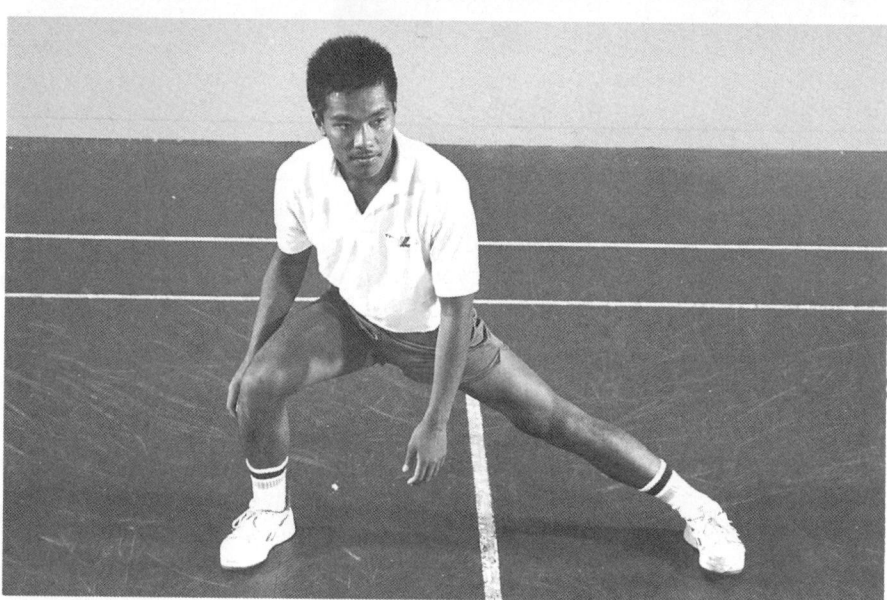

    the other leg to be stretched. Repeat with the other leg. Hold each stretch for 20 seconds.
5. Touch your toes for 20 seconds. This is more effective if done in a sitting position but can be done standing.
6. Step sideways with one foot, keeping your feet 3 to 4 feet apart. Bring your hips and torso over one leg to stretch your groin muscles. Repeat to the other side. Hold each stretch for 20 seconds.
7. Begin a slow rally to warm up while playing. You can start your rally while jumping up and down (as if you were rope jumping). This helps your legs get ready for the more forceful contractions you will have to make in the game.
8. Take your racket and practice imaginary shots—first slowly then faster.
9. Rally with a partner.

Checklist for the Warm-Up

1. Warm up your muscles by jogging around the gym, doing jumping jacks, or jumping or running in place. Next, swing your arms in big circles, forward and backward.
2. Slowly stretch your muscles, holding each stretch for at least 20 seconds. Stretch your
   a. hamstrings by touching your toes.
   b. groin by taking a long sideways step and bringing your torso over one leg.
   c. torso by twisting slowly right, then left.

Cooling Down

After you have played, don't just shake hands and sit down, or your muscles will tighten. A cool-down reduces later muscle soreness and helps eliminate the build-up of waste products (such as lactic acid) in your body. Take a short walk, or do some of the stretches that you did for your warm-up. The idea is to allow your muscles to gradually relax and cool down.

Summary

1. The grip is very important. Without the proper grip for the chosen stroke, you will drastically reduce your chances of making an effective shot.
2. The ready position is similar to that used in many other sports. It should allow the player to move quickly in any direction.
3. Always have your racket up and ready so that you can take the offense.
4. The home-base position is in midcourt and slightly forward of the midpoint of the centerline.
5. Good footwork is essential in badminton.
6. Always warm up adequately for your rally or game.
7. Cool down after the game to reduce the chance of muscle soreness.

CHAPTER 5

Service and Service Return

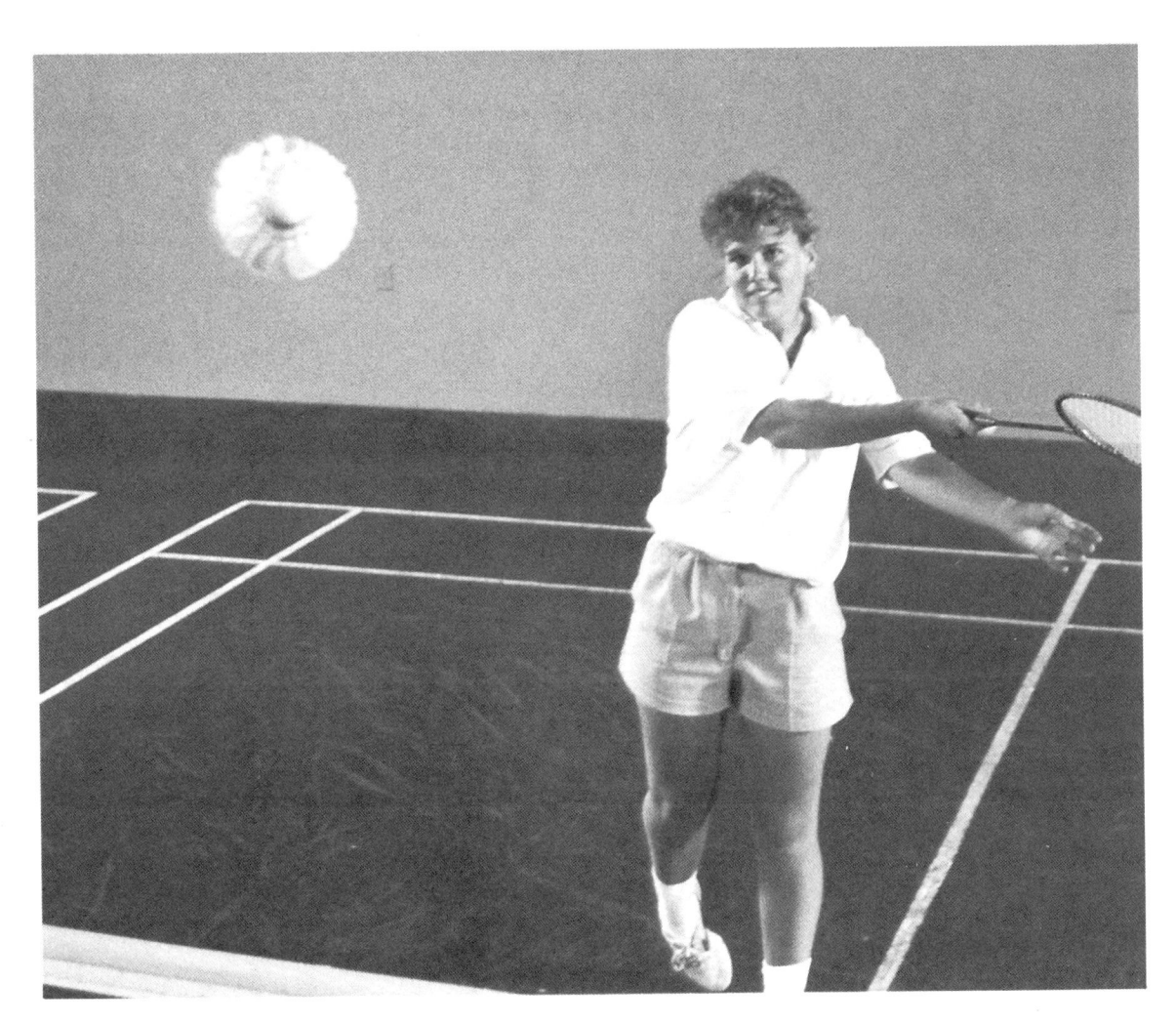

Outline

The Serve
    High, Deep Serve
Checklist for High Deep Serve
Short Serve
Checklist for Low, Short Serve
    Flick Serve
    Drive Serve
    Backhand Serve

Checklist for Low, Backhand Serve
Service Return
    Singles Returns
    Doubles Returns
Serving and Scoring
Summary

The Serve

The serve should be learned first, since all rallies start with one. Also, it is through the serve that a player begins to "control the point."

The rules state that, when serving, you must stand in the service court, and your feet must both stay in contact with the floor until after the shuttle is hit. During your arm action, your racket must contact the shuttle below your waist, and the entire head of your racket must be below your hand.

High, Deep Serve

The high, deep service is used primarily in singles play. If not hit by your opponent, this serve should land as close as possible to his or her opponent's back line. The objective is to move your opponent deep into the back court.

Take a position approximately 2 to 3 feet from the front service line and close to the centerline. (The point where the center line meets the front service

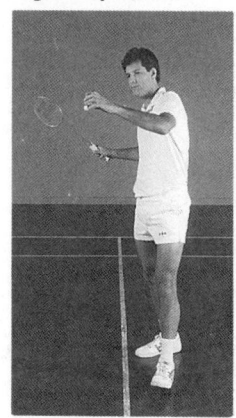

High deep serve:

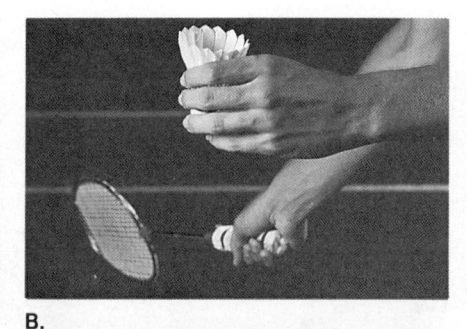

A.
B. 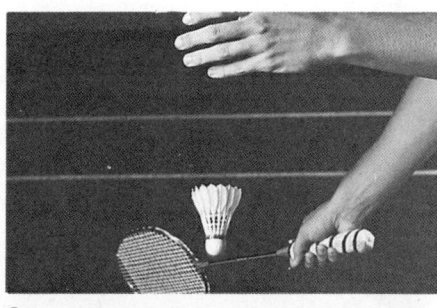
C. 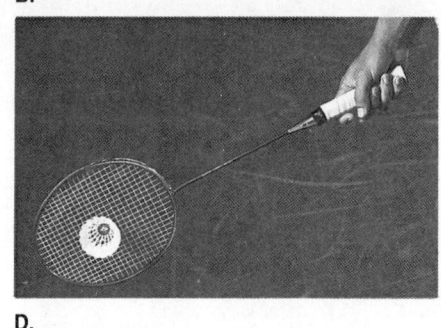
D. 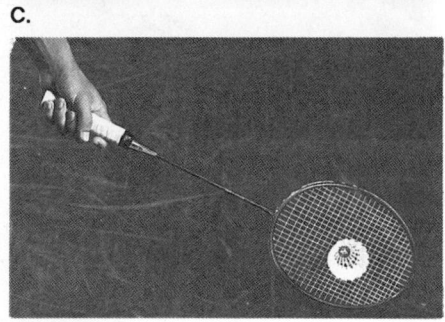
E.

A. Two to three feet from T
B. Fingers gripping shuttle at base, racket ready
C. Drop shuttle
D. Contact (right)
E. Contact (left)
F. Follow-through

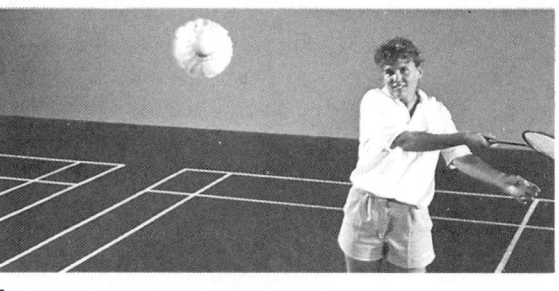

F.

High deep serve

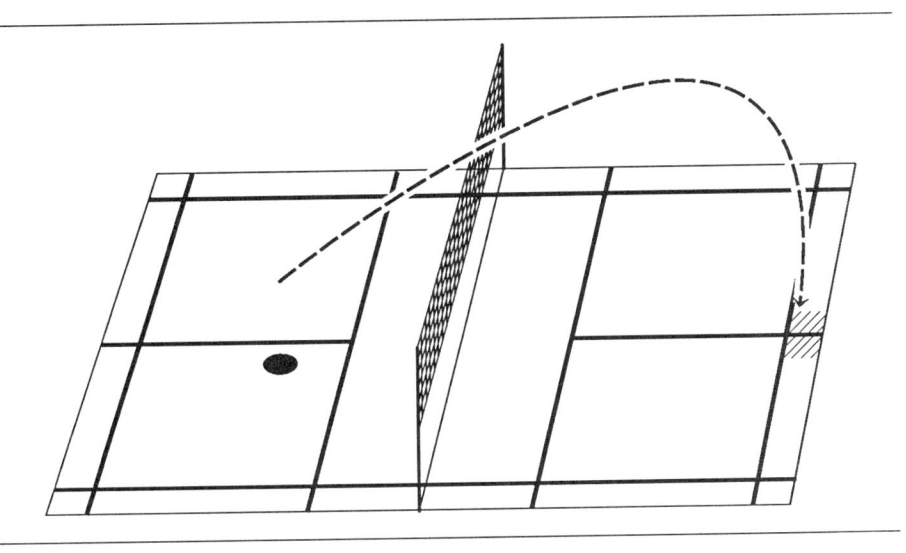

line is often called the "T.") Stand with your feet comfortably apart (about shoulder width), with your racket-side foot back (the right foot for right-handed players). Your knees should be slightly bent.

Hold the shuttle by its cork base between the thumb and the index and middle finger of your left hand. Extend your left arm outward in front of the right shoulder. This allows you to hit the shuttle near waist level and in front of you. Many beginners tend to hold the shuttle low, near waist level, then drop it. This forces them to hit it at too low a point. You always want to hit the shuttle at as high a point as is legally possible.

Your right wrist will be cocked up and back so that the racket head will be raised and the wrist will be at or above waist level. Your weight will be on your rear (right) foot.

As you drop the shuttle in front and to the side of your body (at about 45-degree angle), your weight will shift forward (to your left foot), and you will swing the racket through the shuttle. At the contact point, the entire head of the racket must be below the level of your hand and below waist level.

Your body rotates in the direction of the shuttle's flight, and your wrist straightens and snaps the racket through the shuttle. You should be hitting up and out.

Follow through over your left shoulder, and let your forearm continue its rotation. Remember that you are not allowed to move or slide either foot until after contact is made with the shuttle.

The only difference in your stance between serving from the right and left courts is that when you are serving from the left, your back foot will be further behind your front foot.

The most common error for beginners is bringing the racket forward before dropping the shuttle. This results in missing it completely—a fault.

Since the shuttlecock is very light and is designed to catch a great deal of air in its flight, it drops slowly. Your racket swing must compensate for this slow drop. So the idea is to drop the shuttle, then hit it after it is already dropping.

Checklist for High, Deep Serve

1. Do I have a forehand grip?
2. Is my non-racket hand extended outward to where the shuttle can be dropped effectively?
3. Is my racket behind my body with the wrist cocked?
4. Did I drop the shuttle before I started the racket forward?
5. Was the shuttle dropped to the racket side of my body?
6. Did I contact the shuttle at about knee height?
7. Did I bring the racket through quickly by using the power of my wrist and forearm?
8. Did I follow through over my non-racket shoulder?
9. Did I hit the shuttle up and out?

Short Serve

The low, short serve is used more often in doubles than in singles. The doubles service court is not as long as the singles service court, so the high, clear serves cannot be hit deeply. But since the doubles service court is wider than the singles court, the short serves can be placed farther from the receiver. In addition, the low serve forces your opponent to hit the shuttle up and gives you the opportunity to take the offensive by hitting the shuttle down.

It takes a great deal of practice to be able to serve the shuttle low over the net and to land it close to the front corners of your opponent's service court. When used in singles it can keep your opponent off balance or bring him or her closer to the net so that the deep serves will be more effective.

Take a position about 2 to 3 feet from the front service line and close to the centerline. Both arms will stay close to your body while your weight rests on your forward foot.

Short service drop:

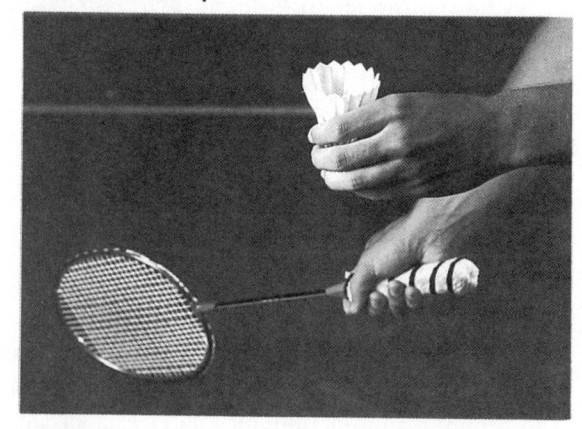

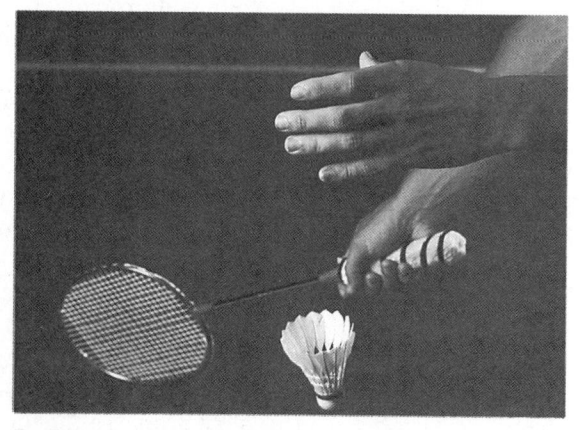

A. Ready

B. Drop

Short service drop (cont'd):

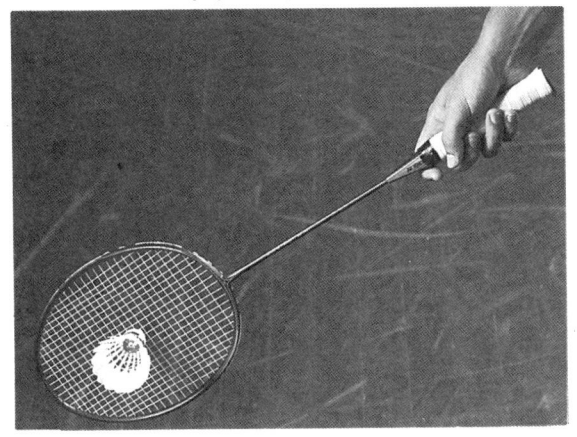

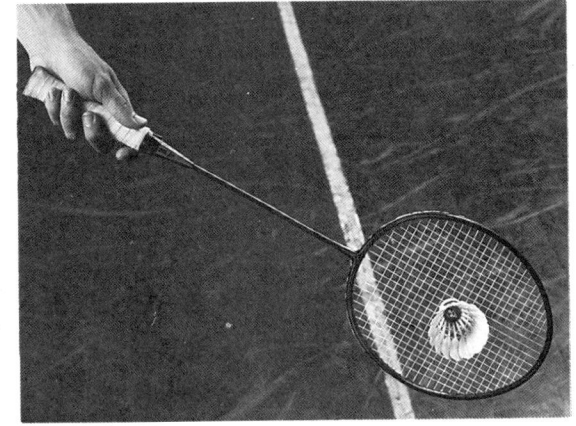

C. Contact (right)

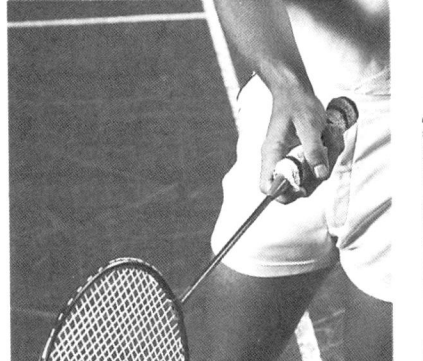

D. Contact (left)

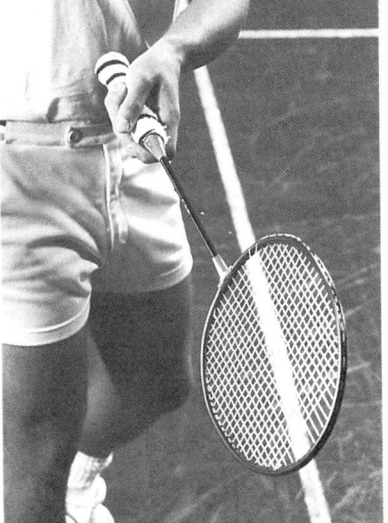

E. Follow-through (right)

F. Follow-through (left)

Drop the shuttle before you start your racket forward. Your wrist will be cocked backward and upward. It will stay cocked throughout the stroke—even during the follow-through. Drop the shuttle in front of, and to the side of, your body, and swing the racket in a nearly horizontal plane around your body—with the racket head just below waist level. The racket head should be angled slightly upward to direct the shuttle just over the net. Gently guide the shuttle forward so that it just clears the net. Beginners should clear the net by 12 inches or less, advanced players by no more than 2 inches. The serve should then fall into your opponent's service area just past the service line. If the shuttle touches the net but still falls into the correct service court, it is a legal serve. The short serves should fall just past the service line. Try to hit either of the front corners of the opponent's service court. The short serve requires a great deal of practice.

Low short serve

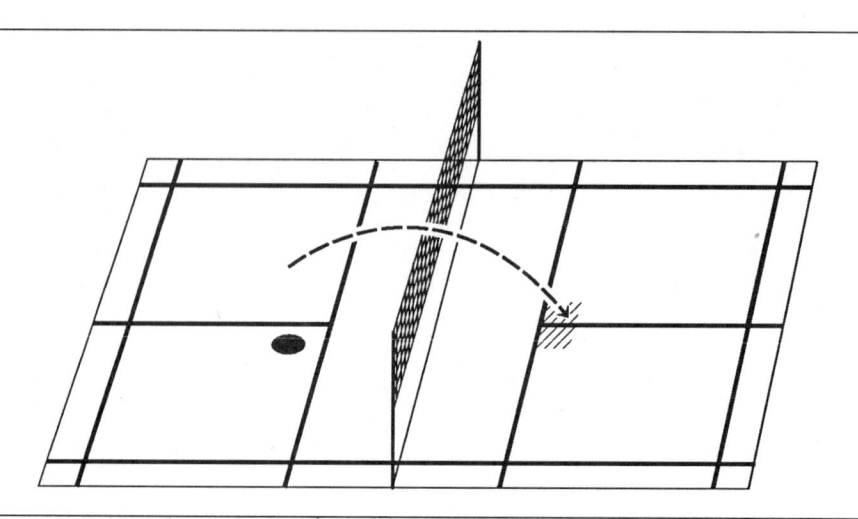

Checklist for the Low, Short Serve

1. Do I have a forehand grip?
2. Is most of my weight on my forward foot?
3. Are my elbows bent and close to my waist?
4. Is my right hand near my right hip?
5. Is my wrist cocked backwards?
6. Did I drop the shuttle before I started my racket swing?
7. Was the shuttle dropped to the front and right side of my body?
8. At contact did my wrist remain cocked?
9. Did I guide the shuttle over the net with my right forearm?

Flick Serve

The *flick serve* is a harder-hit serve with a low trajectory, just high enough to clear the outstretched racket when your opponent is reaching up to return it. It is used in both singles and doubles—most often in doubles, when your opponent often rushes your short serve.

The shuttle is dropped in front and away from the body. The flick serve should look just like a short serve, except that as the racket nears the shuttle, its speed is accelerated to drive the shuttle to the back court by uncocking the wrist. If the serve is not returned, it should land deep in your opponent's back court.

Drive Serve

The *drive serve* is hit hard, but lower than a flick serve. It is used more often in doubles, when your opponent is expecting a short serve. Doubles teams that play a side-by-side alignment may find it especially valuable because it can force a weak return. Beginners may occasionally use this serve in singles, but advanced players do not, because it is easy for the advanced opponent to reach and cut it off.

SERVICE AND SERVICE RETURN 39

Flick serve:

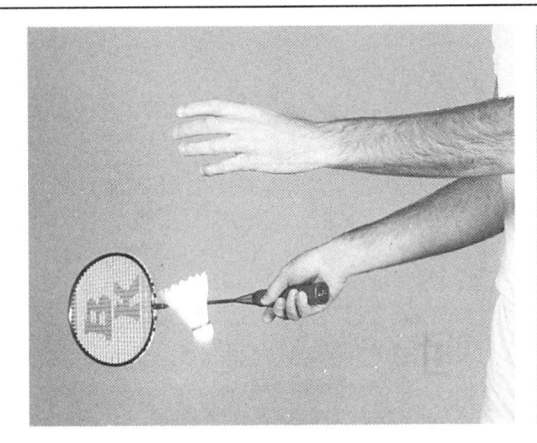

A. Drop

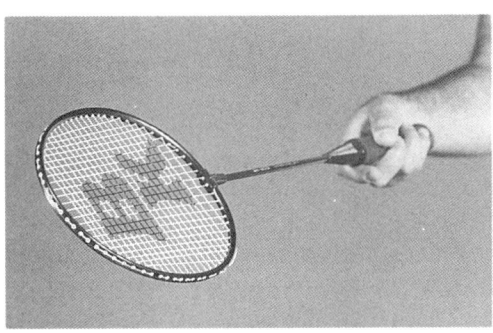

B. Contact

C. Follow-through

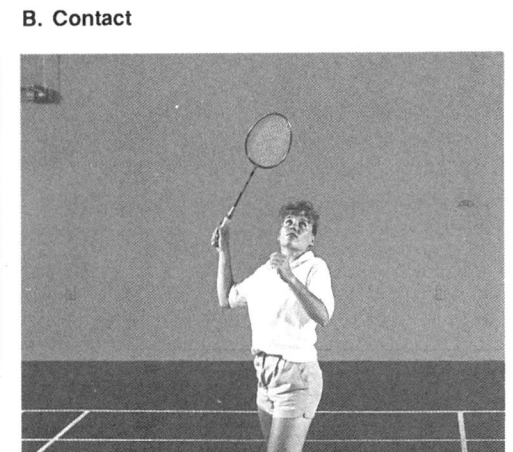

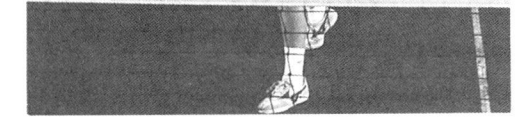

D. Speed of shuttle accelerates drive into opponent's back court

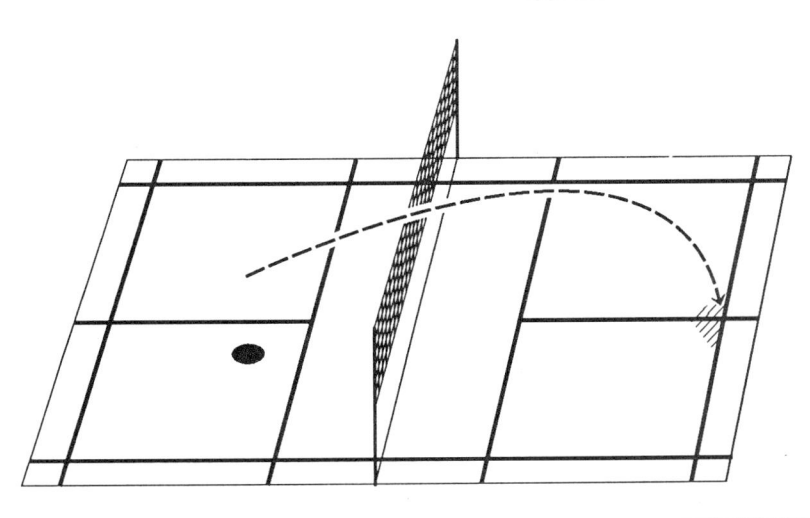

Drive serve

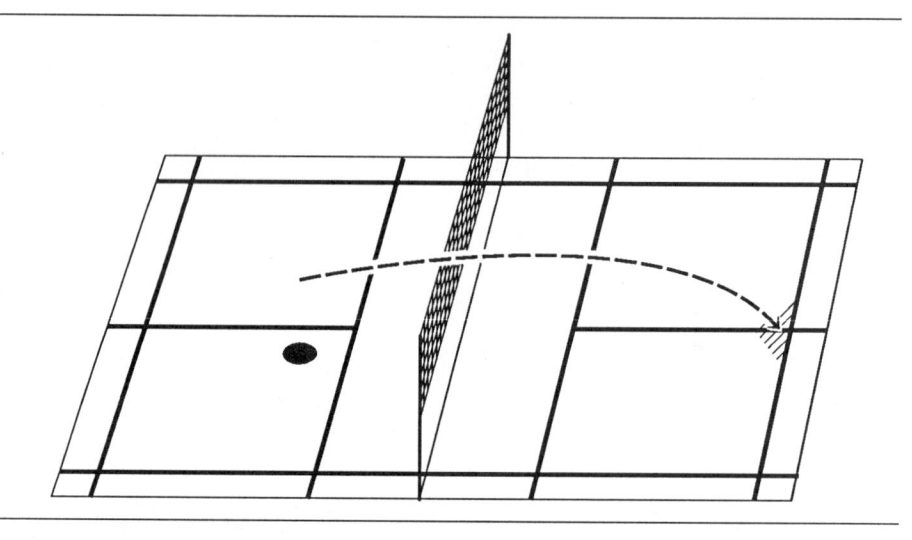

Backhand Serve

The *backhand serve* is used in doubles as a more effective method of serving the low short serve. It was developed in Indonesia in the 1960s and is now becoming popular in the western countries. In this serve there is very little backswing, and the shuttlecock is hit just after it leaves the hand. Consequently, it takes less time to clear the net, giving your opponent less time to adjust to your serve. Also, because the white shuttle blends in with the white clothing of the player, it is more difficult for the receiver to see.

For this serve your stance will be parallel to the net. (When your shoulders and an imaginary line touching the front of the toes on each of your feet are parallel to the net, your stance is parallel. Some players will only have their

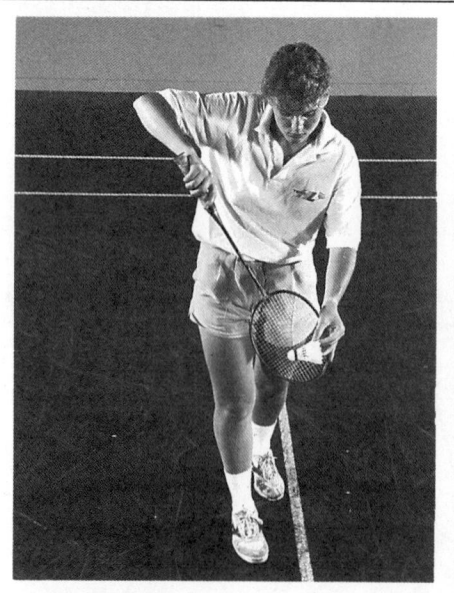

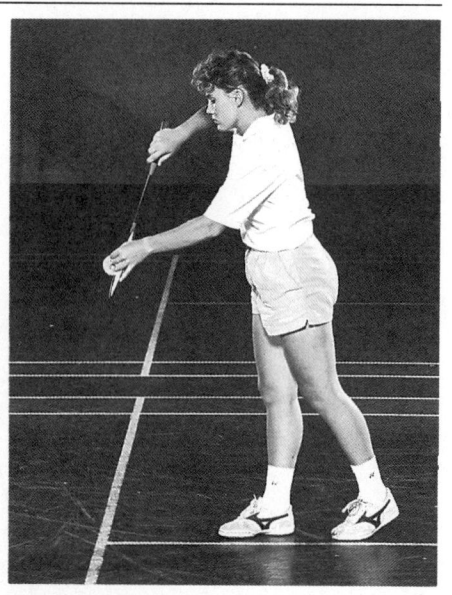

Backhand serve:

A. From front　　　　　　　　**B. From side**

Gripping shuttle for backhand serve

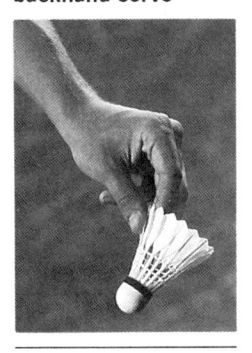

racket-side foot forward.) Your grip will be the true backhand grip, with your thumb behind the racket handle.

Thumb and index finger should lightly grip just one or two feathers of the shuttle, holding it just below your waist and parallel to the face of the racket. (Some people like the racket face perpendicular to the floor; others like the face opened toward the ceiling. Whichever racket position you choose, the shuttle should be parallel to the racket face.)

Your right elbow will be shoulder-high, and your right arm will be away from your body. Your forearm and racket extend at a 45-degree angle downward. Remember that the shuttle has to be hit below the waist to be legal. It should just barely clear the net, landing close to your opponent's serve line.

For variation, this serve can be hit harder and become a flick or a drive serve.

How to hold racket for backhand serve:

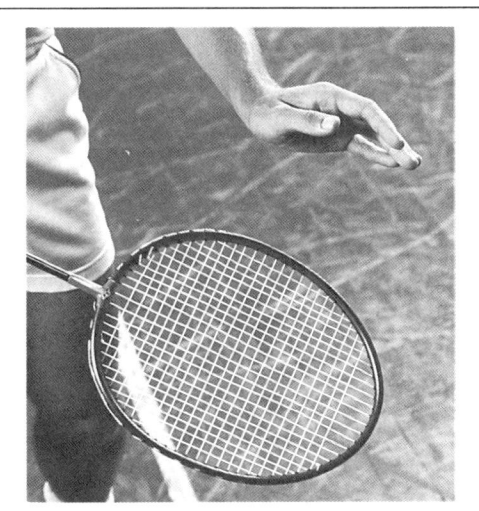

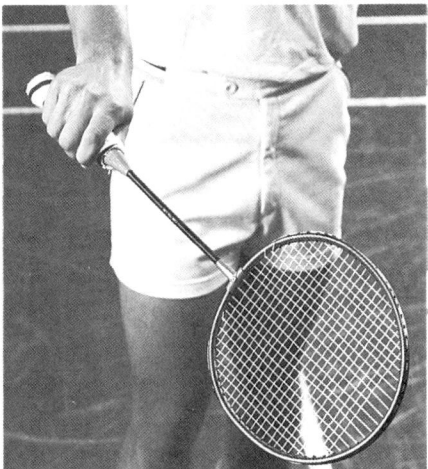

A. Parallel to floor

B. Perpendicular to floor

Checklist for Low, Backhand Serve

1. Do I have a backhand grip with the thumb behind the handle?
2. Is my grip higher on the handle—away from the base?
3. Is my stance parallel to the net?
4. Am I holding the shuttle below my waist and by the tip of the feathers?
5. Is my racket-arm elbow shoulder-high and away from my body?
6. Is the racket head angled down behind the shuttle?
7. Did I "push" the shuttle over the net?
8. Did the shuttle start dropping before it passed to the other side of the net?

Service Return

Your body position for the service return is as follows: left shoulder and foot forward, feet spread about 2 feet apart, with most of your weight on your forward foot so that you can move backward more quickly, and knees and ankles flexed, with weight on the balls of your feet. Your torso is flexed forward, and your racket is held up above your head and ready to hit.

Singles Returns

Your position on the court will be slightly forward of midcourt and slightly to the backhand side of your service court. To return a singles serve, you would be a bit deeper. From the left court, you will be the same distance back but closer to the center of the service court—the midline between the sideline and the centerline. Your alignment should allow you to protect your backhand so that you have a greater chance of playing the return with a forehand.

Watch the shuttle before it is served, and be alert for any possible serve. Then get to it as quickly as possible in order to catch it at its highest point. Hitting lazy underhand returns puts no pressure on the serving team.

On short serves, quickly lunge forward to the net. Your best choices of a return shot are: (1) a drop to the front corner away from your opponent or (2) a high clear. On the deeper flick serves, jump back quickly, and hit a drop or a smash.

Your best strategy is to place your shot in an area of the court that forces your opponents to play defense. Use high clears to the backhand corners and drops along the net. The most effective types of returns are

- Clear return.
- Attacking clear return.
- Smash or half-smash.
- Drop return.

Singles service return:

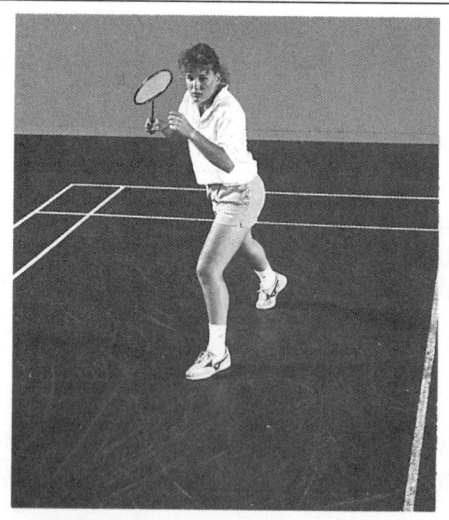

A. Right court   **B. Left court**

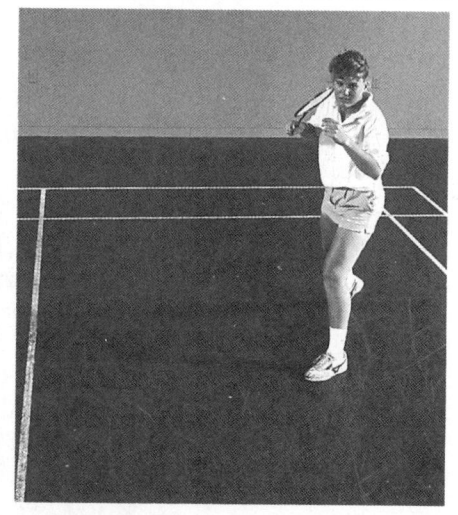

SERVICE AND SERVICE RETURN 43

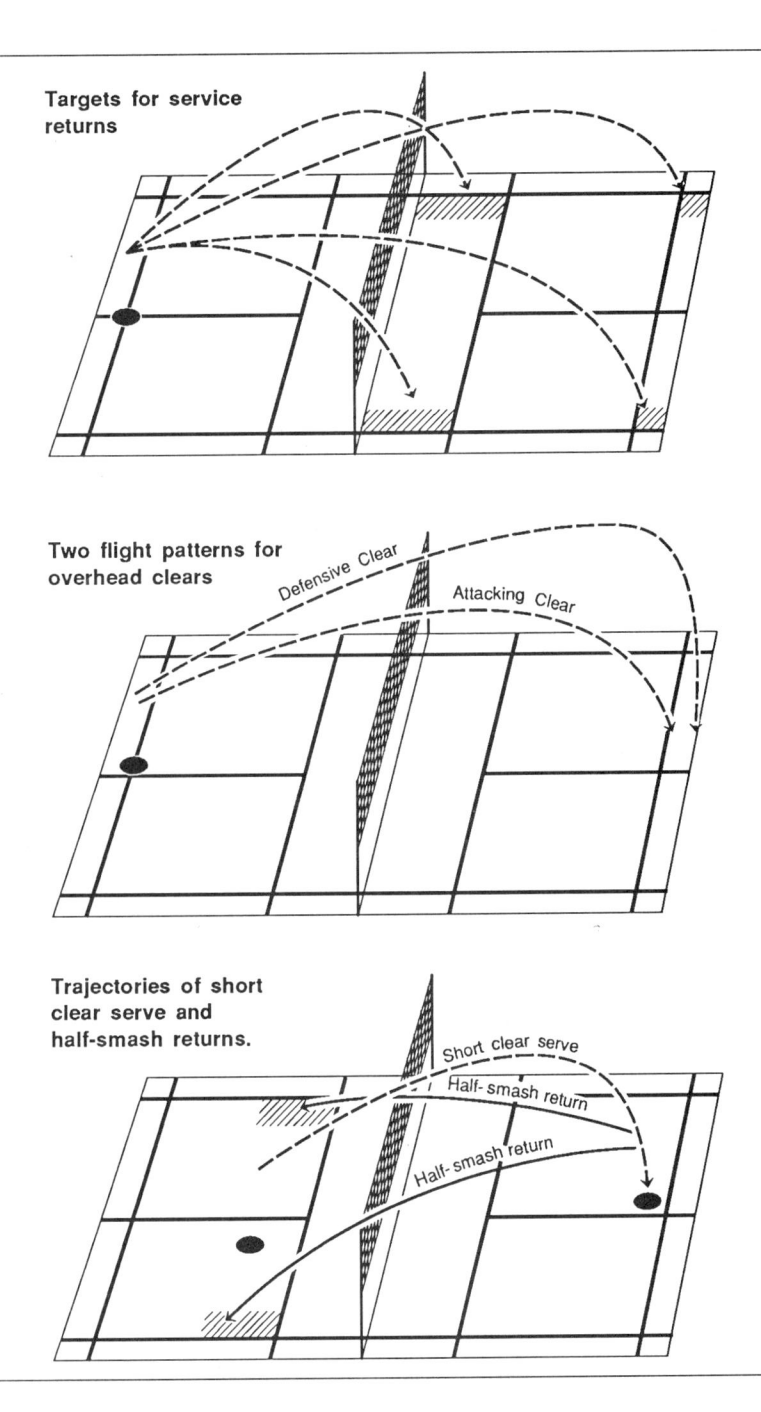

Targets for service returns

Two flight patterns for overhead clears

Defensive Clear

Attacking Clear

Trajectories of short clear serve and half-smash returns.

Short clear serve

Half-smash return

Half-smash return

The *clear return* (also used in doubles) is a high shot that clears the opponent and lands just inside the back line. Keep it away from your opponent, preferably to the backhand side. Make your opponent move. This is especially effective if you have been hitting drop returns, leading your opponent to anticipate another drop and thus come to the net. As with other clearing shots, you will need a strong wrist action and a follow-through along the intended line of flight.

Drop return

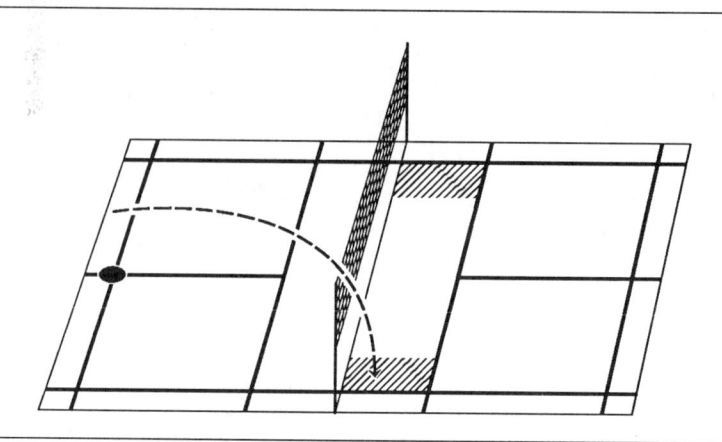

The *attacking clear return* can be used if the opponent has hit a high, weak serve and is close to the net. The trajectory in this return is lower, so the opponent has less time to react to the shot. It is aimed just like the regular clear return. The danger in this return is that if the opponent is quick to react, he or she can cut the shuttle off and smash it.

The *smash* or *half-smash return* can be used when a clear serve is too short or too low. It puts your opponent on the defensive by forcing an upward hit.

The *drop return* can be used anytime you want to move your opponent away from the center position. If your opponent has hit a drop serve, you can counter with an underhand drop return close to the net.

Doubles Returns

Stand within a foot of the front service line and within a foot of the center service line. This will allow you to attack the low serve quickly and force your opponents to play defense.

Unless you find it very successful, don't rush to the net on your return too often. While you may occasionally guess correctly that your opponent is hitting a short serve, your opponent may also catch on to your strategy and catch you off-guard with a high serve.

Your return strategy should be to force your opponent deep with a clear, or to hit down so that your opponent must hit up with a defensive shot. The most effective returns are

- Drop return.
- Clear return.
- Half-court pushes down the middle or to the sidelines (into the alley).
- Harder pushes or drives down the middle or to the deep corners.

Vary your returns to keep your opponents off-balance.

The *doubles drop return* must be very close to the net and close to the near sideline as it is returned to your opponent. (Unless your opponent is out of position, do not hit this shot crosscourt.) This is because in doubles your opponents will usually play one person up and one back. The person close to the net will therefore have a better chance of smashing it back if it is hit high. Consequently, you have to hit lower and wider in doubles than in singles.

SERVICE AND SERVICE RETURN   45

Position for doubles return:

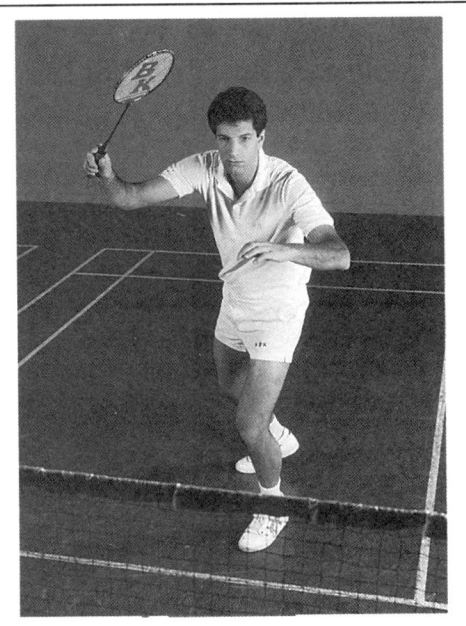

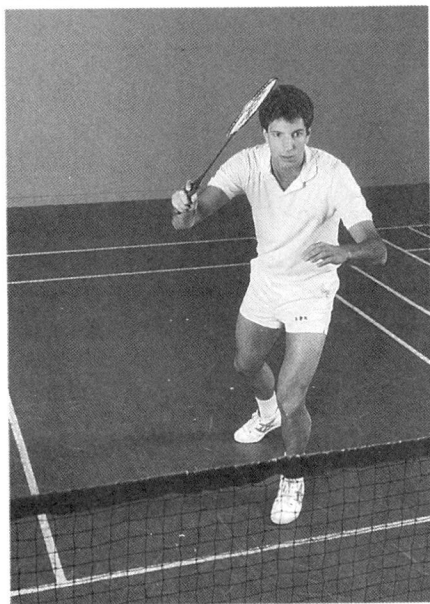

A. Right court

B. Left court

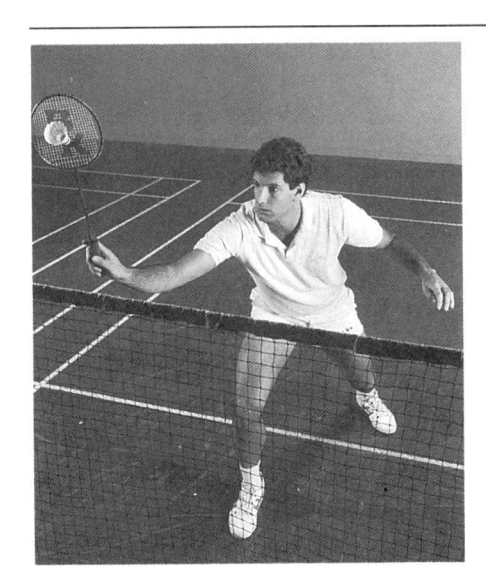

Short service return attack in doubles

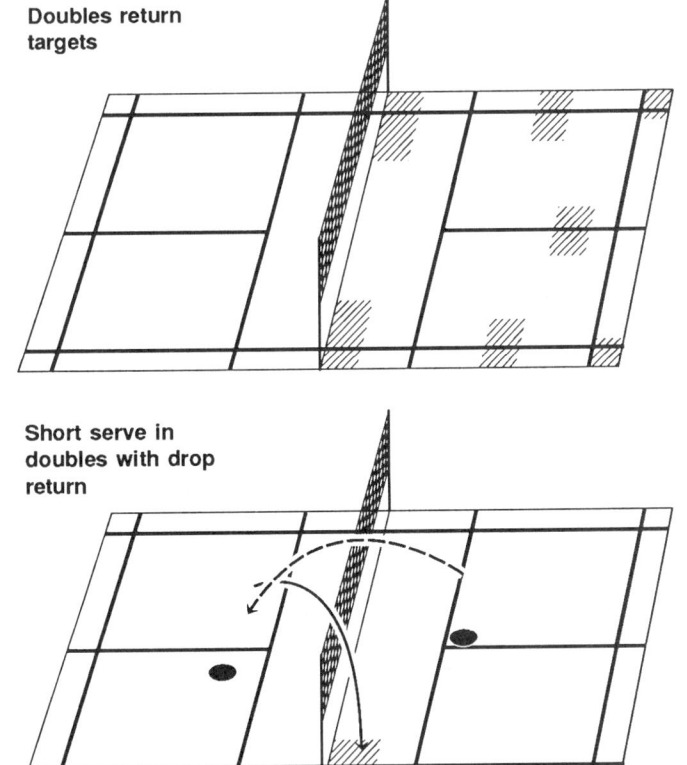

Doubles return targets

Short serve in doubles with drop return

Short serve with doubles return drop

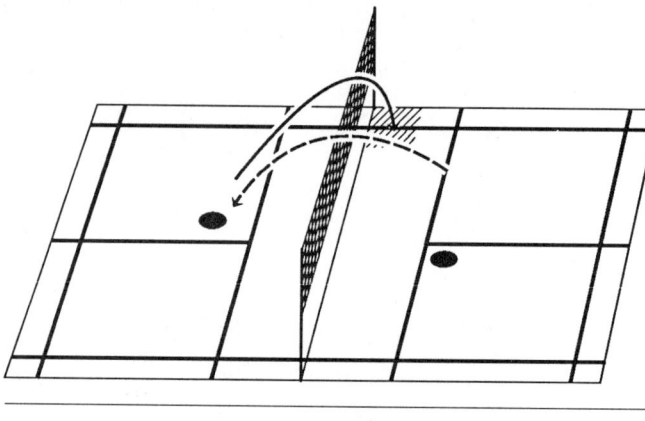

Target trajectory for half-court push return

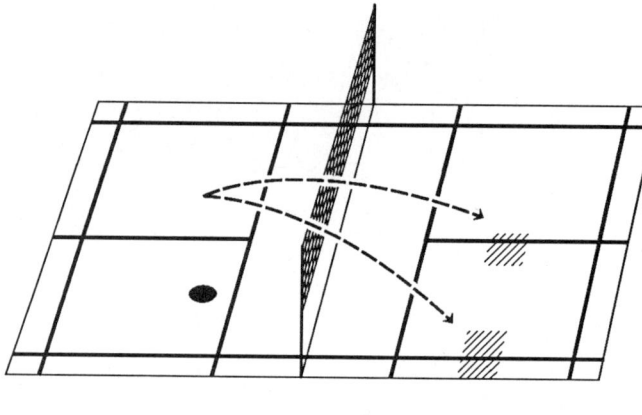

Doubles drive return

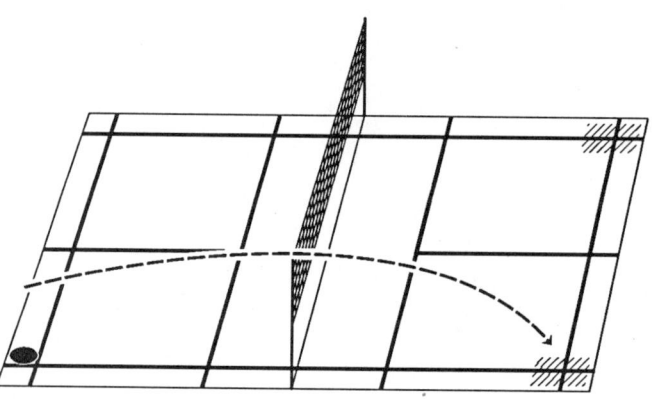

The *clear return* is the same as in singles.

The *halfcourt push return* is a difficult shot because it must be played nearly perfectly or your opponents may gain the advantage. When placed correctly, it will fall low behind the net player and force the back player to hit up.

The *doubles drive return* is hit along the sidelines with a short, fast backswing. It is used if your opponents are playing up and back and should always be hit straight down the near sideline.

Contact the shuttle in front of your body and within 2 feet of the net. It is hit flat, with the racket head parallel to the net. Only the wrist is used in this shot.

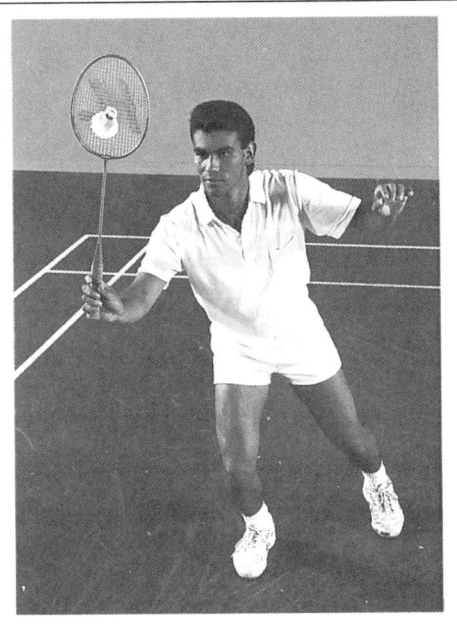

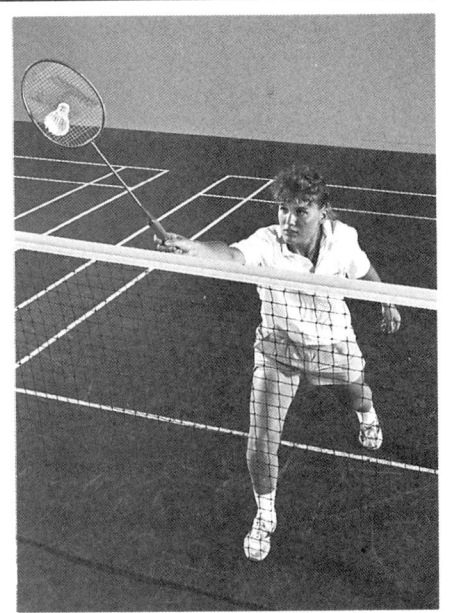

Doubles drive return contact   **Push return contact**

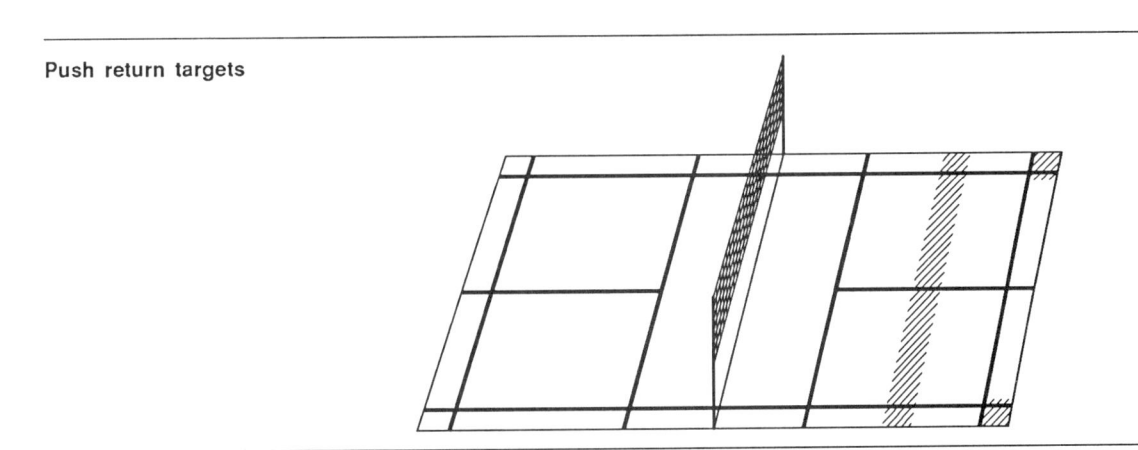

Push return targets

If it is a backhand shot, make certain that your thumb is behind the handle in a good backhand grip.

The *push return* is a nearly sidearm return (backhand or forehand) that is pushed with the forearm into the deep backhand corner, deep forehand corner, or into your opponent's body. It starts downward from your racket.

Serving and Scoring

In badminton only the server can score points. The receiver must win a rally in order to be able to serve and then have an opportunity to score.

In singles the serve is from the right service court whenever the server's score is an even number. The serve is from the left court whenever the server's score is an odd number. Remember that the service court for singles is long and narrow and that the sideline is the inside court boundary.

In doubles the serving team will always start an inning with the server in the right service court serving first. If the serving team wins the point, the same server moves to the left court and serves. The server keeps alternating courts until the serve is lost by a fault. (See Chapter 3.)

When the first server has lost the serve in the first inning of play, the service is over, and the opponents serve. The team that serves first in doubles keeps the serve only as long as the original server continues to make points. (After the very first inning, each player continues to serve until there is a fault.)

The opponents' first server will serve from the right court. If a point is made, he or she will move to the left court. Courts are alternated until the first server has lost the serve. The second server will then serve from the same court in which he or she was standing when the serve was lost. In other words, one cannot serve twice in a row to the same receiver. After the starting team has lost the service, the second team serving is allowed to have each server serve until the point is lost.

Once the original receivers have both lost their serves (called *two hands down*) the team that served first in the game will regain the serve. This time each player on that team must lose his/her serve before the other team gets another turn at serving.

A simple way to remember who should serve first in an inning is to remember which side of the court you were in during your team's first serve. You should be on that same side whenever your team's score is zero or an even number. You should be on the other side of the court whenever your team's score is an odd number.

The *rally* begins once the shuttle is served legally over the net, and it continues until one team has made a fault. If the serving team faults, the partner then takes the turn.

Once you begin to play, you will realize the importance of position, footwork, and strategy.

Summary

1. Only the person serving can score points, so the serve is very important.
2. The basic serves are the clear and the short, but a flick serve or a backhand serve can also be used. In singles the high, deep serve is most often used; in doubles, the low, short serve. The drive serve is a change-up serve that can be very effective as is the flick serve.
3. Whether playing singles or doubles, mix up your serves.
4. In singles the server serves from the right court whenever the server's score is an even number—0, 2, 4, etc. The server serves from the left court whenever the score is an odd number—1, 3, 5, etc.
5. In doubles the first inning allows only one player to serve. That player serves first from the right court and alternates sides with each point won. When the other team gains its serve, the server in the right court serves until his or her team has committed a fault. Then the partner serves. After each point the server alternates courts.

CHAPTER 6

Overhead Strokes

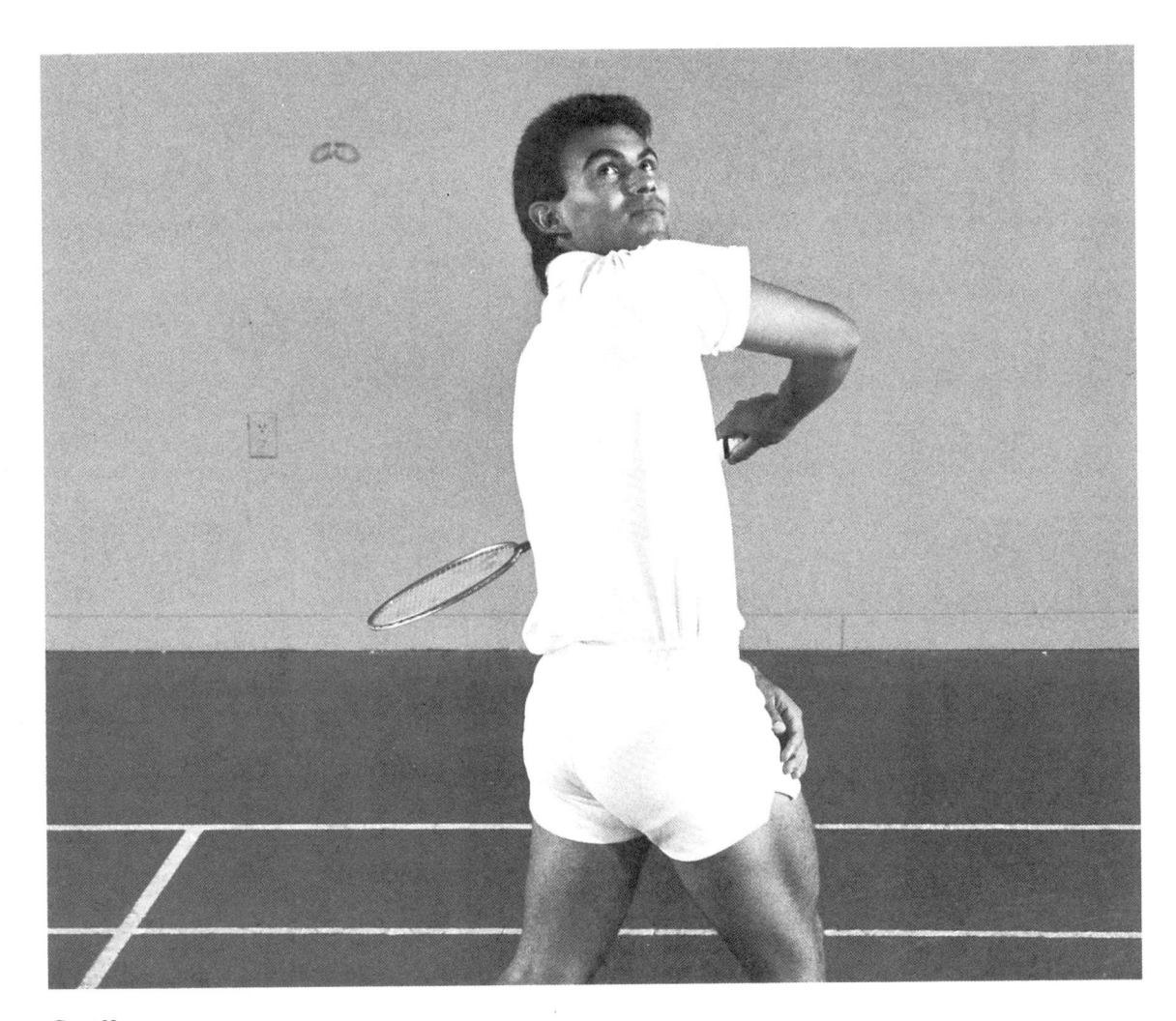

Outline

Forehand Overhead Clear
Throwing Drill for Beginners
Backhand Overhead Clear
Attacking Clear
Smash
Checklist for the Smash
Half-Smash

Drop Shot
Checklist for the Drop Shot
Push or Dab Shot
Drive Shot
Round-the-Head Shot
Summary

The overhead strokes that are absolutely essential for any badminton player are the clear, the smash and half-smash, drop, dab or push, and the drive.

These are the "fun" strokes. There are very few service aces in badminton. Most of the points come from rallies. Since the net is 5 feet high, you will want to hit most strokes above your head. This way you have the option of hitting downward hard or hitting a controlling shot that places the shuttle quickly in an area difficult for your opponent to cover.

If you are forced to hit underhand, your choices are limited, allowing your opponent to control the game. To be in control, you must play an attacking game by hitting as many overhead shots as possible, forcing your opponent to hit up or to hit from deep in the backcourt.

Basic overhead strokes:
A. Topview

B. Sideview

OVERHEAD STROKES

The fundamental overhead strokes for beginners are
- Forehand and backhand clears and drops.
- Forehand smash.

The intermediate-level overhead shots are
- Drives.
- Round-the-head shots.

The advanced overhead shots are
- Backhand smash.
- Attacking clear.
- Half-smash.

Forehand Overhead Clear

The *forehand overhead clear* is used mostly in singles to move an opponent to the back court. Take a forehand grip; then, from your base position, watch the oncoming shuttle and get into position behind it, with your right shoulder in line with it. Bring your racket up and behind your shoulders with the racket head pointing slightly downward. This is often called the *back-scratching* position because the racket head is nearly touching your back. Get into this position quickly. If you hit the shuttle while you are moving backwards, you are not getting back and behind the shuttle quickly enough.

When you hit this shot, your left shoulder should be closest to the net and your left arm extended and pointing up at the shuttle. Your weight will shift to the right leg as you prepare for the shot and take your backswing, then shift to the left foot as the stroke is taken.

Forehand clear:

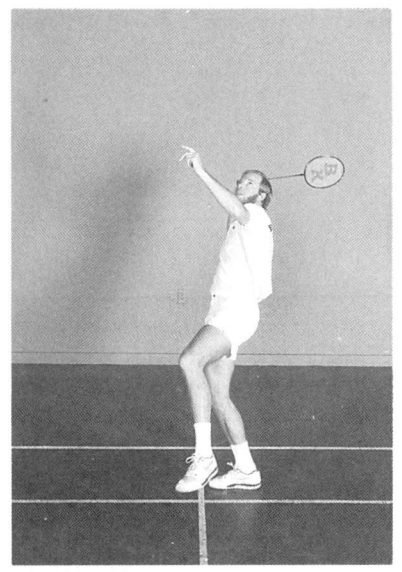

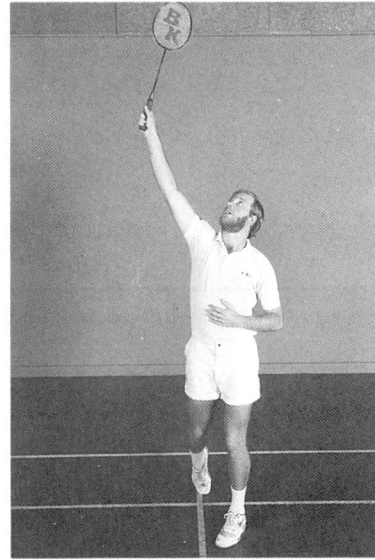

A. Backswing   **B. Foreswing**

Forehand clear (continued):

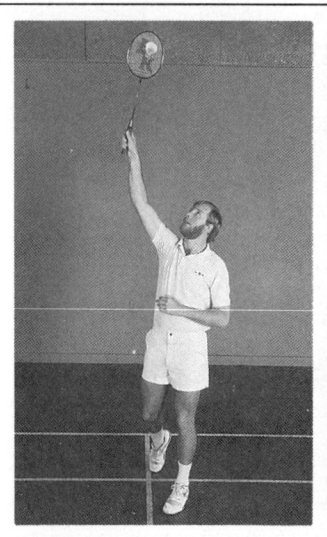

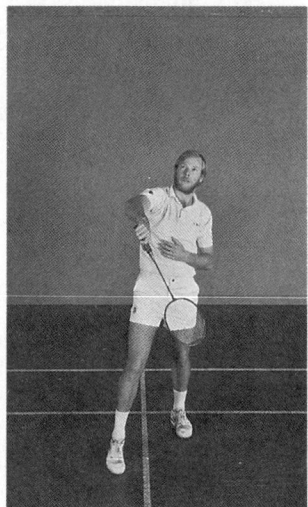

C. Contact

D. Follow-through

Bring the racket up to meet the shuttle as high as possible. The shuttle is contacted above and in front of your shoulder, not out to the side. It is hit at the highest point possible. At contact, your arm straightens, and your wrist snaps quickly. The racket head will be facing upward slightly at contact. Let the racket continue outward and to the left side of your body. When you shift your weight to your forward foot, keep your forward knee slightly flexed for balance.

The overhead clear shot should drop perpendicular to the floor and land between the baseline and the long doubles service line. This deep shot, which drops straight down, is more difficult for your opponent to hit. If you have time, look at your opponent's feet to see if they are near the baseline, which is a good indication that your clear is deep.

You will note that the shuttle does not follow the same path as a ball would follow. A ball will follow an arc path—with the angle of ascent and descent approximately the same. The shuttle, because it is so light and has great air

Checklist for the High Clear Shot

1. Are you in the ready position?
2. Do you have a forehand grip?
3. Are you behind the shuttle with your left shoulder pointing to it?
4. Is your racket pointed downward behind your back with your wrist cocked?
5. As you swing upward do you contact the shuttle in front of your body with a hard wrist snap, hitting the shuttle high?
6. Do you follow through completely?

almost immediately slow down, then drop nearly straight down. Because of its unusual flight path, beginners often have trouble anticipating where the shuttle will drop.

A good clear will also give you more time to get back to home base (in the center of your court) and will make it more difficult for your opponent to smash effectively, because one cannot smash effectively from deep in one's court. Remember to return to your home base and be in your ready position after each shot.

When you can hit the clear consistently you may want to play a *long and short game.* In this game you will try to keep your opponent back most of the time while occasionally hitting a drop shot to break his or her playing rhythm.

Throwing Drill for Beginners

To learn the arm action for overhead strokes, follow this drill. Start without your racket. Your intention is to throw the shuttle up and out as far as possible. This throwing action is very similar to that used in hitting the clear or the smash.

Turn your body, and face the sidelines with your left shoulder toward the net. With your left foot forward (for right-handers) and weight on your back foot, take the shuttle in your right hand and hold it at the base. Bring your right elbow to shoulder height and away from your body. Your hand and the shuttle should be behind your right ear. Your wrist should be flexed toward the thumb side of your hand. Now throw the shuttle *up and out* as far as you can reach.

Transfer your weight to your forward (left) foot as you release the shuttle. Your upper torso will rotate to your left as your arm comes upward and forward. Try throwing a few more times to get the overall sensation. Check your release

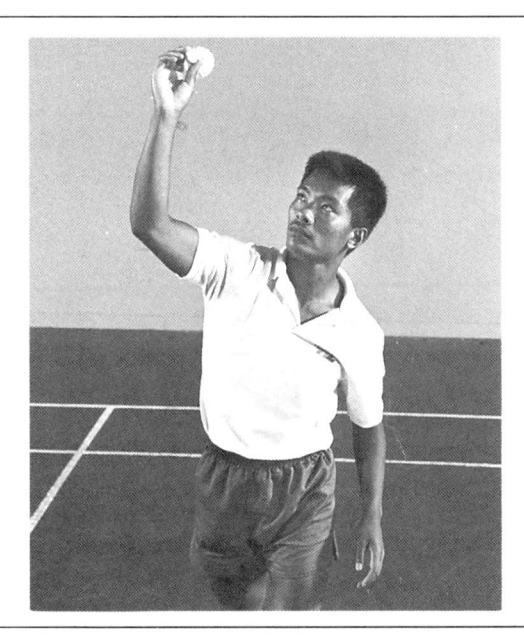

Throwing drill

Try throwing a few more times to get the overall sensation. Check your release in relation to your body with your best throws. This is the angle at which you want your racket to contact the shuttle.

Practice hint: Occasionally while rallying have the opposite player let the shuttle drop so that you can see if it lands near the baseline. This is where a good defensive clear should fall.

Hint for advanced players: In order to get back to the center of the court quickly, advanced players should "scissor" their legs as they hit the high clear shot. In this technique the weight is shifted from the racket-side leg to the other leg as the shuttle is hit. The player gets under the shuttle, jumps upward from the racket-side leg, and then, after hitting the shuttle, lands on the other leg and moves forward toward the home-base position.

Backhand Overhead Clear

The *backhand overhead clear* is used mainly in singles when the player cannot get in position to hit a forehand. Always make the forehand shot if possible. For the backhand clear you must turn your body completely to the backhand side so that you are facing your left sideline. Your right shoulder should be toward the net and your right foot pointed diagonally toward the left net post. Your elbow should be pointing at the oncoming shuttle. The shuttle should be away from the body so that a circular swing can be made. (This is different from the forehand clear, which is hit directly over the shoulder.) This shot will require more backswing from the shoulder because the muscles in the back of the forearm (which supply the power for backhand shots) are not as strong as those in the front of the forearm, which supply the power to forehand shots.

The shuttle is contacted high and in front of your body. Your weight will shift to your right foot as you hit and follow through.

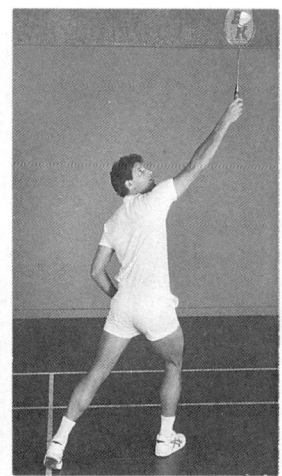

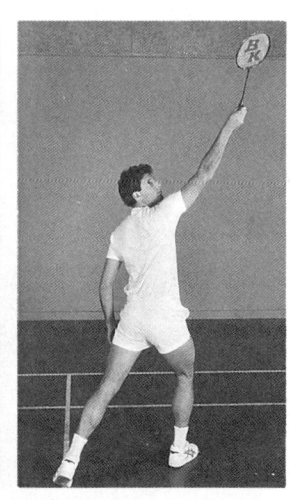

Backhand clear:

A. Backswing   **B. Foreswing**   **C. Contact**   **D. Follow-through**

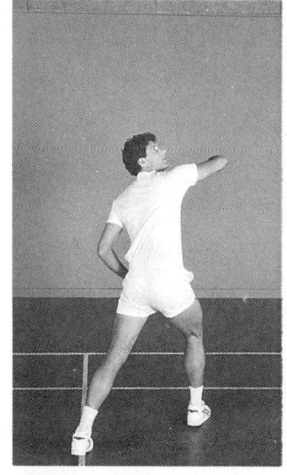

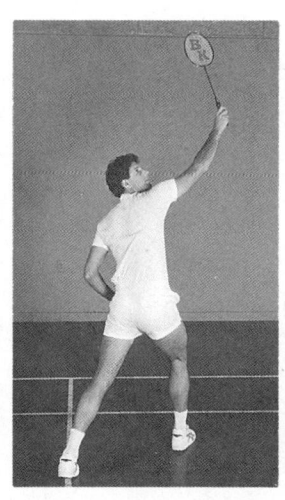

Attacking clear:

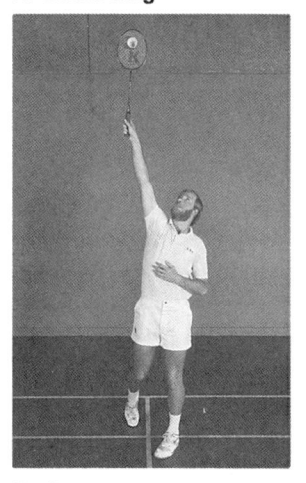

A. Backswing 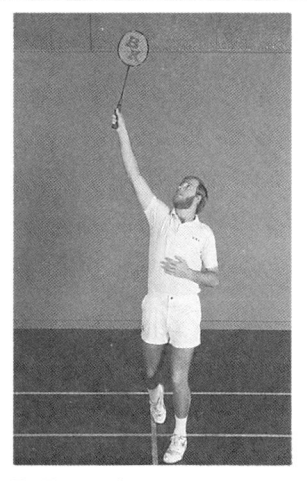   B. Foreswing

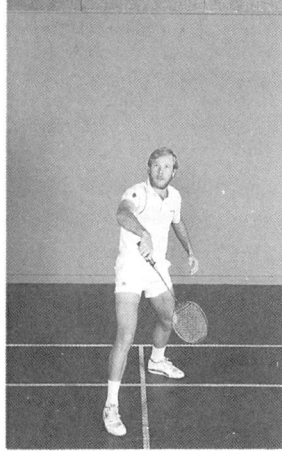

C. Contact   D. Follow-through

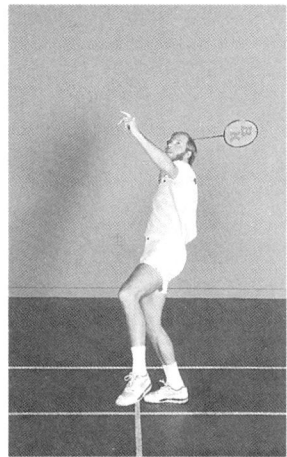

Attacking Clear

The *attacking clear* is used when your opponent is close to the net, and you think you can get the shuttle over his or her head for a winner. It is hit like a clear except that the trajectory is lower.

Smash

The *smash* is the most powerful stroke in badminton. It is hit extremely hard and, if hit effectively, usually ends the rally. However, speed is not always as important as the downward angle. Body position is the same as for the clear, the difference being in the angle of the racket at the contact point. In the clear the racket head is pointed up, while in the smash it is angled down. A second difference is the increased speed of your forearm and wrist snap.

As you get set for the smash, your left shoulder should be closest to the net. The shuttle should be ahead of your hitting shoulder—much farther ahead

Footwork for scissors kick in smash

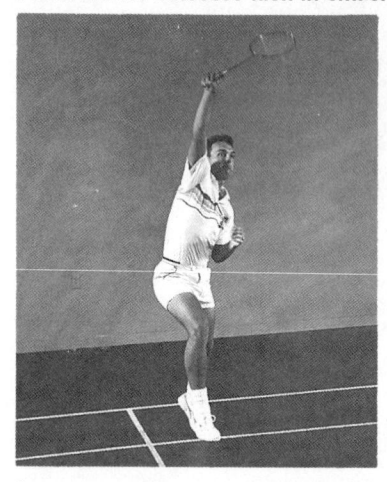

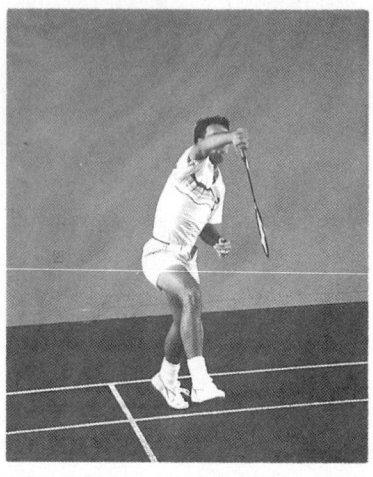

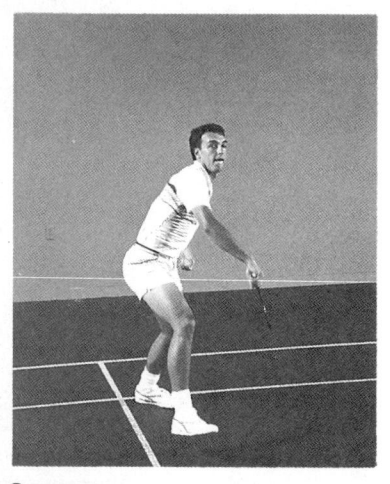

A.   B.   C.

Backhand smash:

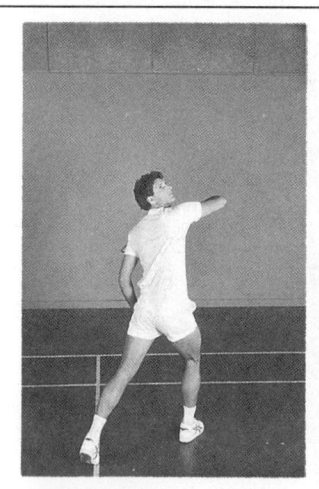

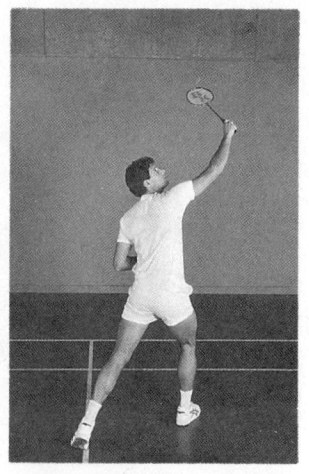

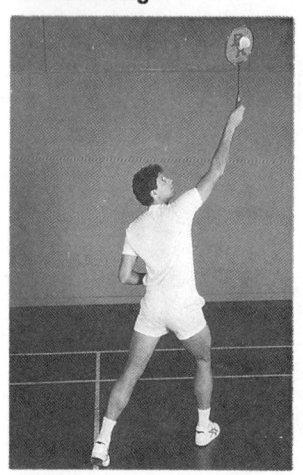

A. Backswing   B. Foreswing

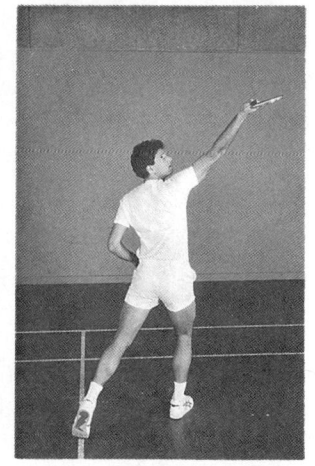

C. Contact   D. Follow-through

than where you contact the clear. (The weaker your wrist, the further forward the shuttle should be hit.) You should hit the shuttle in front of your shoulder and at the highest point possible. Your shoulder, forearm, and wrist will rotate rapidly forward as the shuttle is contacted. Hitting it slightly ahead of your body will give you a greater sharpness of angle on the shot.

As you hit the smash, your upper body should move forward and downward. This facilitates power and follow-through. If you are behind the middle of the court, your forward momentum helps you to get back into the home-base position more quickly and get set for a possible return.

The smash should land near either sideline and at approximately mid-court—10 to 16 feet from the net.

Use this shot only when you expect it to be a winner. Since you are expending a great deal of energy, and you may be off-balance after your follow-through, it is important that it be done effectively.

The smash should be used only when you are in the front three-quarters of the court unless you are a very strong player. Beyond that area your opponent will probably have time to return it, because the shuttle will lose speed as it flies the greater distance, and your opponent can see the shuttle for a longer period of time. But if you have a chance to hit a smash when you are in the forecourt area, there is a very good chance that it will be a winner.

If you find that you are smashing into the net, it means that either you are hitting the shuttle too far in front of you or that you have an exceptionally strong wrist snap. In either case, move under the shuttle a bit more, so that it is not so far in front of you before you hit it. If you are hitting out of bounds, you will need to hit the shuttle farther in front of your body or use more wrist snap.

The smash is probably the most overused stroke in the game—especially among the younger players. The best strategy is almost always to move your opponent up and back, side to side, and wait patiently for the opening for a smash that will be a winner and end the rally.

You can occasionally hit a smash at your opponent's body. The chest-to-hip area on the racket-side of your opponent is most vulnerable to this type of shot.

Checklist for the Smash

1. Are you facing the right sideline?
2. Is your racket pointed down behind your back in the backswing?
3. Do you swing high, then contact the shuttle in front of your body with a hard, downward wrist snap?
4. Do you shift your weight to your left foot as you complete a full follow-through?

Half-Smash

The half-smash is an attacking stroke used in singles, doubles, and mixed doubles. It is hit similarly to the smash, but placement rather than speed is the essential. The power will come more from the wrist snap than from the whole body.

This shot provides a good change of pace. It is essential to place it to the side of the court and with a sharp downward trajectory so that your opponent cannot reach it.

The halfcourt smash, which lands about midcourt, is often more effective than the full smash, which may land deep in your opponent's backcourt. Actually, both shots should be used. When you play both, you keep your opponent guessing as to whether to move up or back to cover your shot.

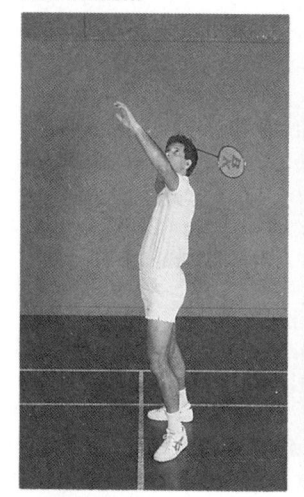

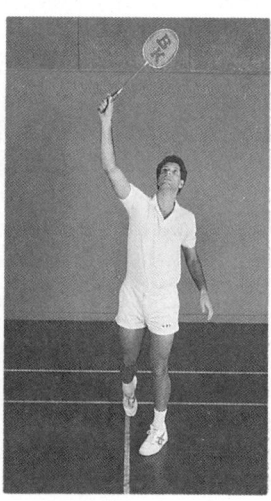

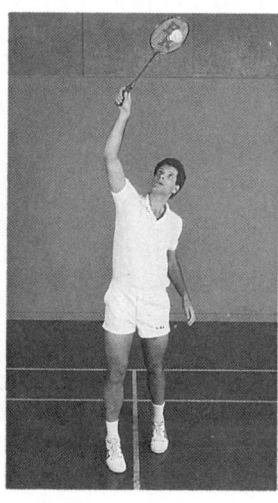

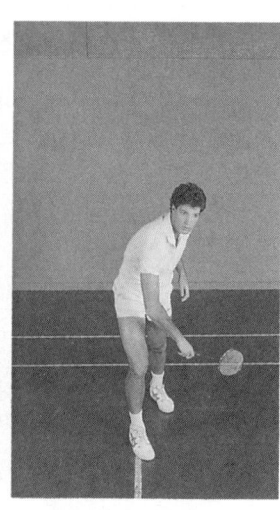

Half-smash:

A. Backswing   B. Foreswing   C. Contact   D. Follow-through

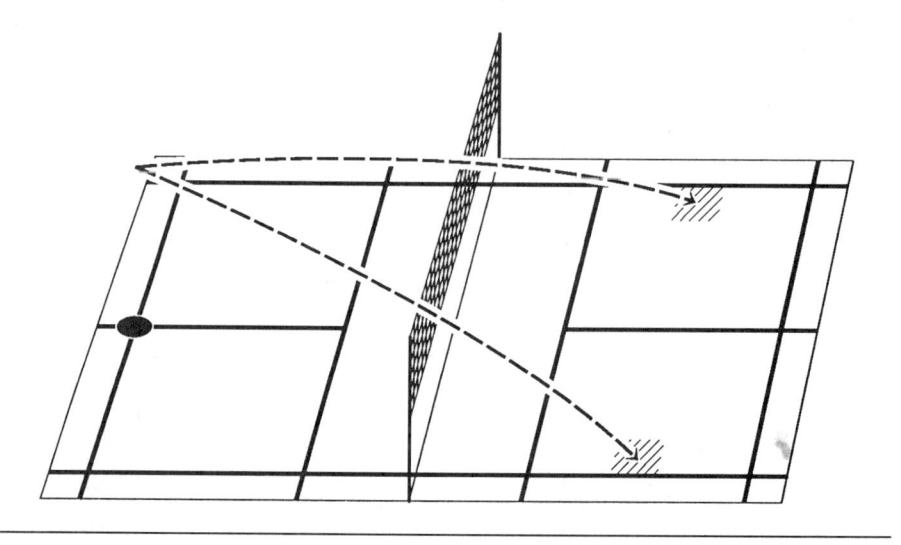

Half-smash trajectories and targets

Drop Shot

The *drop shot* is a soft shot that barely clears the net, then lands close to the net on the other side—preferably in one of the front corners. It is used to move your opponent forward and to force an upward return that may give you the opportunity for a smash shot. It can be used effectively when your opponent is deep or expects a smash.

The arm action for the drop shot should look like the clear—and vice versa—so that you can disguise your shots and thus surprise your opponent. Use the combination of clear and drop to move your opponent back and forward. This will cause fatigue and will often keep him or her off-balance. Remember that deception is the key.

In the drop shot, the shuttle is contacted in front of the body and the speed of the racket at the time of the hit is greatly slowed compared to the clear. The racket head should be perpendicular to the floor or slightly past the perpendicular.

Drop shot:

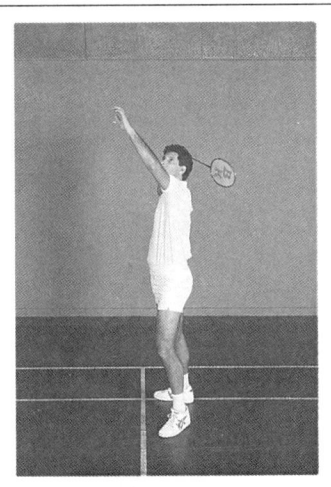

A. Backswing

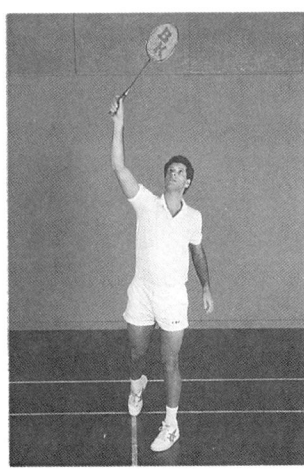

B. Foreswing

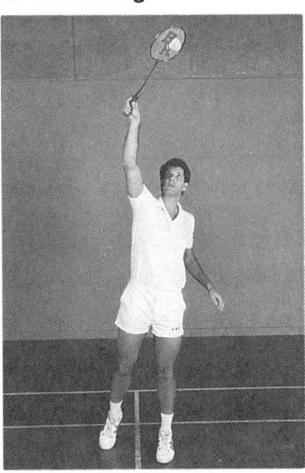

C. Contact

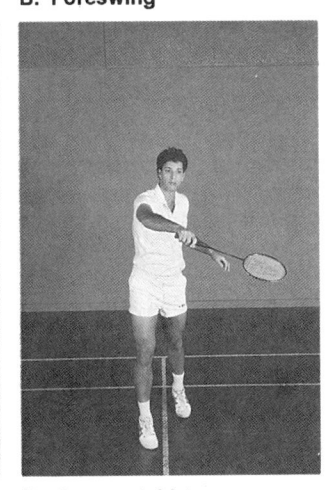

D. Contact (side)

Drop shot

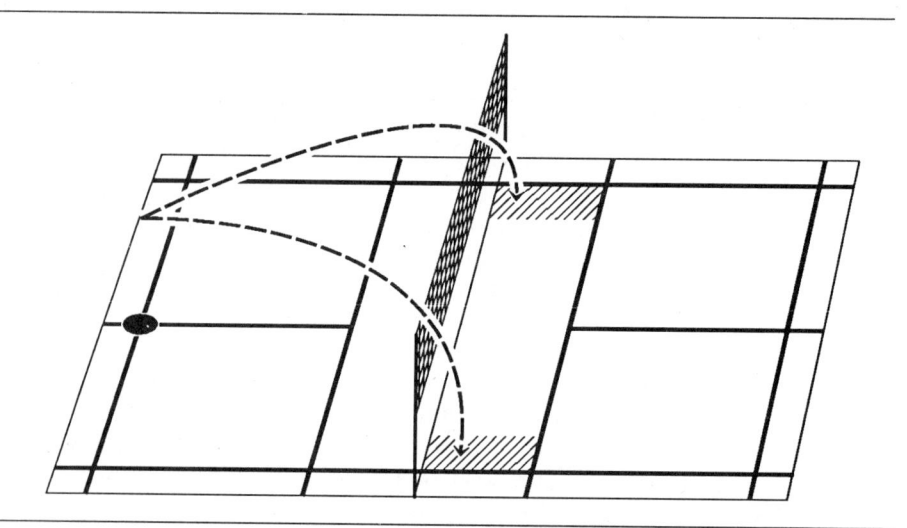

The swing speed should start fast to look like a clear or a smash, but the elbow and wrist snap should be slow as you softly guide the shuttle over the net with your follow-through. If you fail to disguise this shot, your opponent will be able to get the jump on you and make an easy play. Many beginners look like the Statue of Liberty—standing motionless during this shot, a dead giveaway.

Rather than arcing up and coming down, the trajectory of the shuttle should start immediately down from the racket and fall into your opponent's forecourt just past the net. The lower you have to reach to contact the shuttle, and the farther you have to hit it, the more you will have to open the face of the racket upward.

Drop shots can be hit very soft and land just past the net or they can be hit harder, dropping a bit farther from the net. The softness of the shot will be determined by how much of the wrist snap you eliminate as you are contacting the shuttle and making your follow-through.

Checklist for the Drop Shot

1. Do you make the shot look like a smash or a clear by swinging up hard?
2. Do you slow the speed of the racket just before contact to greatly reduce the wrist snap?
3. At contact, was the racket perpendicular to the floor?
4. Do you gently guide the shuttle over the net with your slow follow-through?

Push or Dab Shot

The *push*, or *dab*, is used at the net, primarily in doubles play. It is more of a sidearm block than an overhead shot, hit downward with little or no backswing. The elbow is flexed and held in front of the body. You lunge at the shuttle with your racket-side leg leading. The wrist does not uncock as you push the shuttle, and the follow-through will be very short. You are looking for placement rather than speed in this shot, the most effective placement being near midcourt, between the opponents, and to the sideline.

Timing is very important on the push stroke, which is used primarily in doubles. It is most effective against a team playing up and back.

Dab:

A. Foreswing

B. Contact

C. Follow-through

Drive Shot

Drive shots are sidearm shots played from either the forehand or the backhand sides. These hard shots travel parallel to the net and are used to hit an opening your opponent has left or to force your opponent to quickly cover side to side.

Forehand drive:

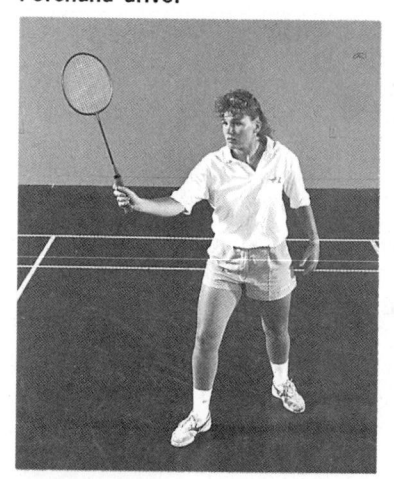

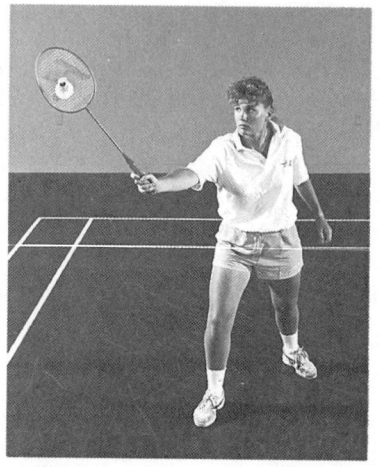

A. Foreswing

B. Contact

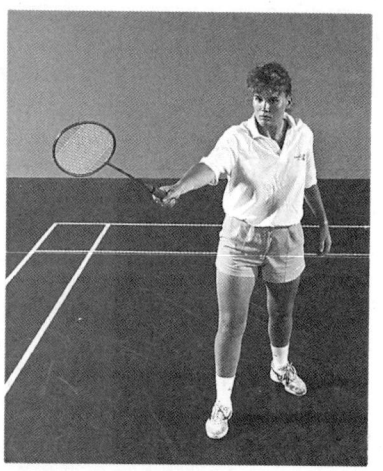

C. Follow-through

Backhand drive:

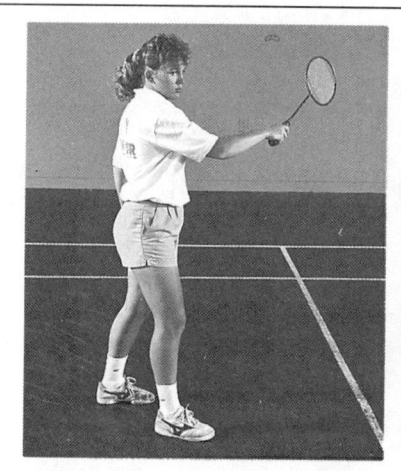

A. Backswing

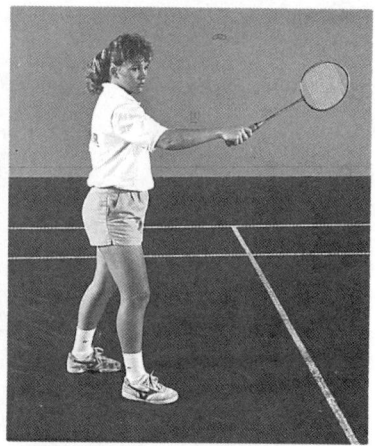

B. Foreswing

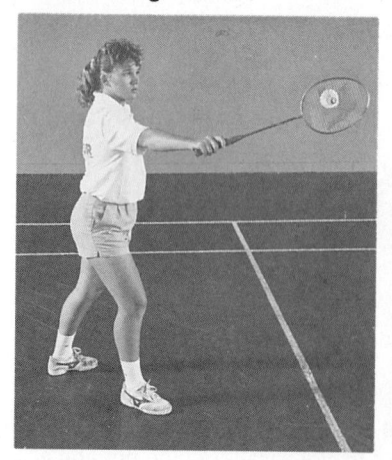

C. Contact

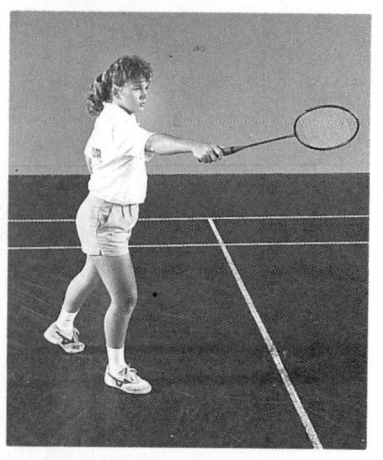

D. Follow-through

For the forehand drive, use your forehand grip and swing in a circular path, whipping your wrist as you contact the shuttle. The contact point is diagonally in front of your left foot. Play it at as high a point as possible so that you will not be hitting up at the shuttle.

Be sure that you are not crowding the shuttle by getting too close. You want to be able to swing freely at it. Your follow-through will be around your body. Your arm and racket will have completed about three-fourths of a circle.

For the backhand drive shot, you use a backhand grip and less wrist but more elbow movement. As you get set for the shot, turn your body so that you are facing the left sideline. Make your backswing with much more elbow bend than in the regular drive shot. Then, with your right elbow pointing at the oncoming shuttle, shift your weight to your right foot as you swing with your shoulders, arm, and wrist. Hit the shuttle in front of you, then follow through around your body.

Your drives can be played down the near sideline or crosscourt—depending on where your opponent has left an opening. Your shots should be hit hard, in a path parallel to the floor—just clearing the net. If your opponent is forced to play your drive while it is still moving fast, there is less likelihood of an effective return. And if it is not played quickly and begins to drop, your opponent will be forced to hit up, giving you the advantage here, too.

Round-the-Head Shot

More advanced players often hit what is called a *round-the-head* shot. Clears, smashes, and drops can all be hit with this stroking action, which is done to avoid having to take a shot on the backhand side (a weaker or a defensive shot). A round-the-head shot allows you to stay on the attack.

Your grip will be a forehand grip—although some players prefer a frying-pan grip. The shot will be made with your body facing the net or while you

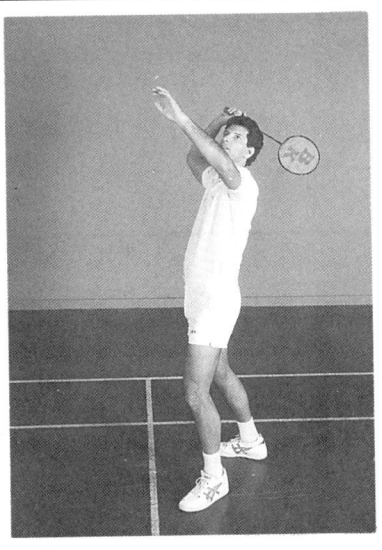

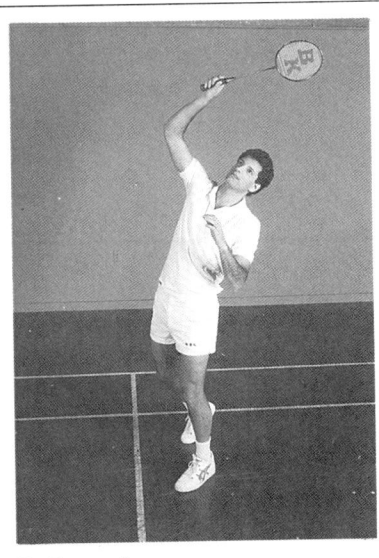

Round-the-head shot:

A. Backswing   **B. Foreswing**

Round-the-head shot: (continued)

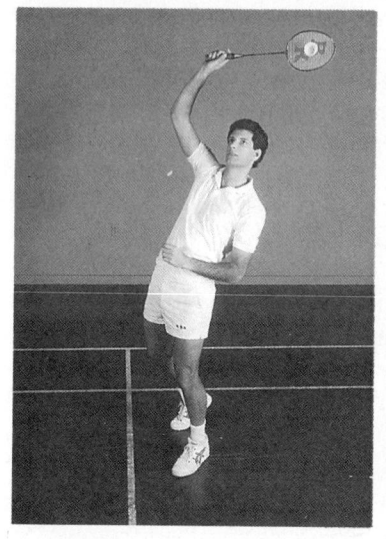

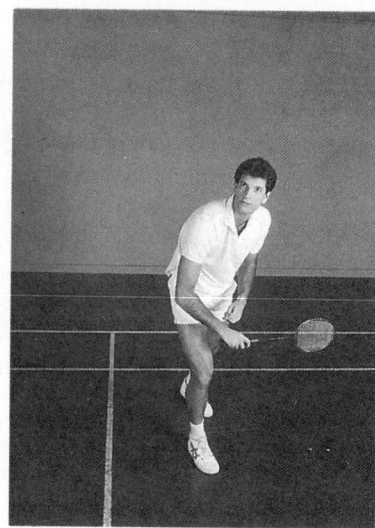

C. Contact

D. Follow-through

are jumping to get better height. The backswing is similar to other overhead shots, but the contact point is above your left shoulder.

If your feet are on the floor, your weight should be on the left foot. If you jump for the shot, you should scissor your legs (a *switch step*), getting your right leg forward, to allow you to get back to your home-base position more quickly.

Summary

1. For all overhead strokes, the direction of the shuttle will be determined by the angle of the racket at the time of contact. So when practicing, concentrate on which racket angle gives you the exact trajectory that you want.
2. Get behind the shuttle as quickly as you can to better enable you to make the kind of shot that you want to make.
3. Always try to take the offense when your opponent hits you a high shot—especially one that is high and short.
4. Always contact the shuttle as high as possible.
5. The major overhead shots are
   - Forehand overhead clear.
   - Backhand overhead clear.
   - Drop shot.
   - Smash.
   - Half-smash.
   - Dab or push.
   - Forehand drive.
   - Backhand drive.
   - Round-the-head shots.

CHAPTER 7

Underhand Strokes and Smash Returns

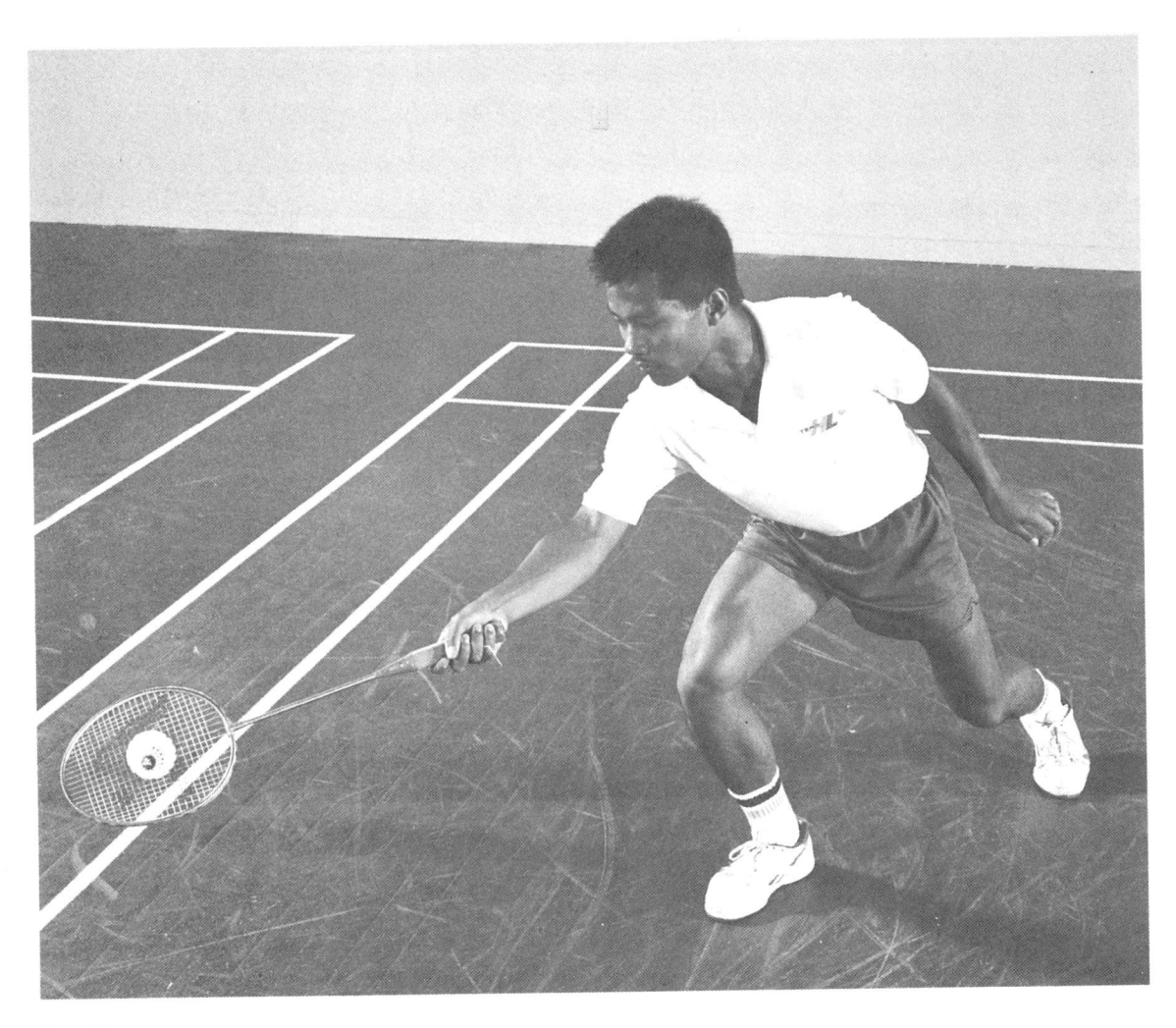

Outline

Forehand Underhand Clear
Backhand Underhand Clear
Checklist for the Underhand Clear
Underhand Drop

Defensing the Smash
Hairpin Drop or Dribble
Checklist for the Hairpin Drop
Summary

While you would prefer to hit all of your shots downward, using overhead strokes, your opponents will often catch you with a drop shot or smash, and then you will have to hit underhanded. In doing so, you will be playing a defensive game. You will therefore want to keep your opponent off-balance by hitting the shuttle deep in a clearing shot or having the shuttle drop close to the net.

The underhand shots are

- Underhand clear.
- Underhand drop.
- Hairpin drop.

As in all badminton shots, you want to hit the shuttle at the highest point possible.

Forehand Underhand Clear

When your opponent makes an effective drop shot into your forecourt, you must go on the defensive—so it is best to hit an underhand clear. This will force your opponent into the backcourt and give you time to get back to your home-base position.

Assuming that the shuttle is dropping toward your forehand side, get to the shuttle as fast as you can. Your first step will be a short one with the

Forehand underhand clear:

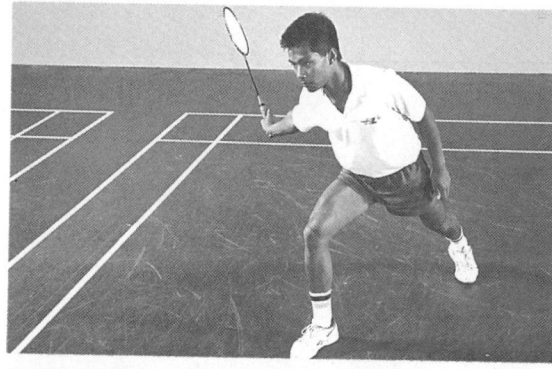

A. Backswing

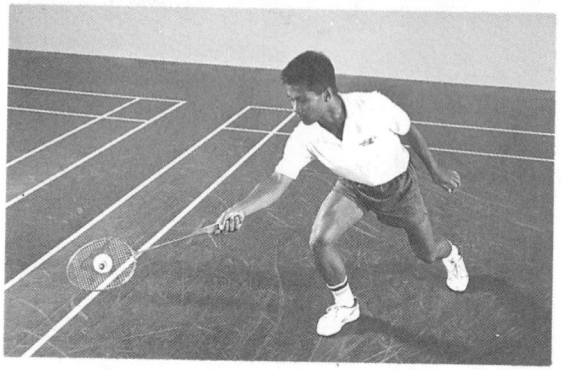

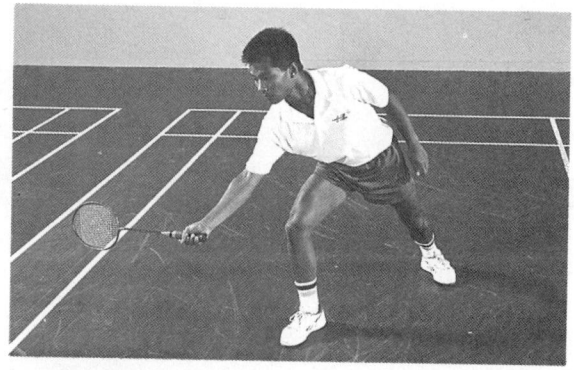

B. Foreswing

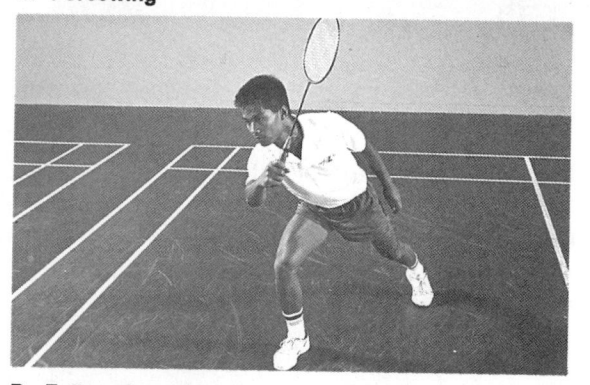

C. Contact

D. Follow-through

left leg. Your right leg should then come forward with a long enough step to bring you to the shuttle.

Reach for the shuttle. Getting too close will inhibit your swing. Bring your racket down and under the oncoming shuttle. Your wrist should be slightly cocked.

Contact the shuttle in front of your body with your weight on your forward foot. Swing the racket upward while uncocking your wrist and whipping it through the shuttle. Follow through in the direction that you intend the shuttle to go. It should land within 2 feet of your opponent's baseline, and its flight should resemble that of a high singles serve.

Remember to step with your right foot. This will extend your reach by about 1 foot. It will also allow you to get back to your home base more quickly to get ready for the next shot.

On crosscourt shots, contact the shuttle harder in order to make up the extra distance it will have to travel.

Backhand Underhand Clear

On strokes made from your non-racket side, change to a backhand grip. Your last step as you reach for the shuttle will be with your right foot. Get to the shuttle as soon as possible. Your racket should be in line with and behind

Backhand underhand clear:

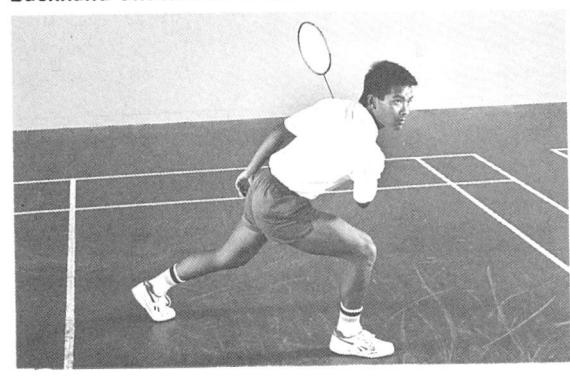

A. Backswing

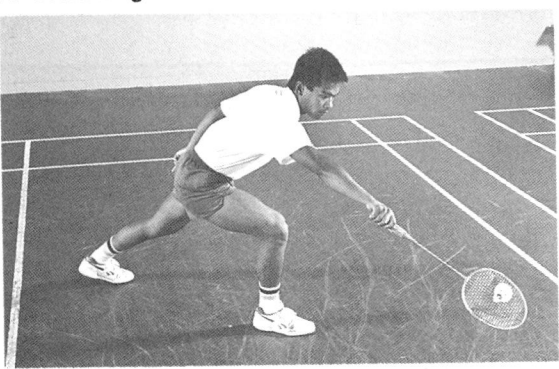

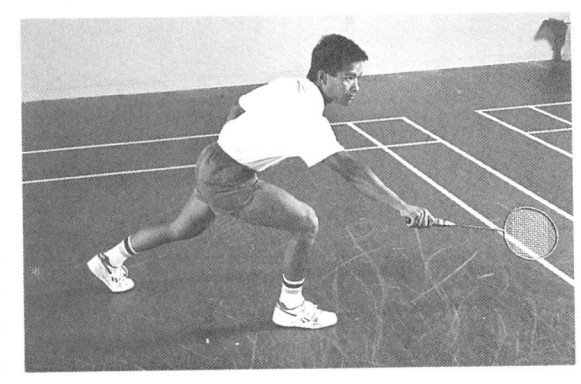

B. Foreswing

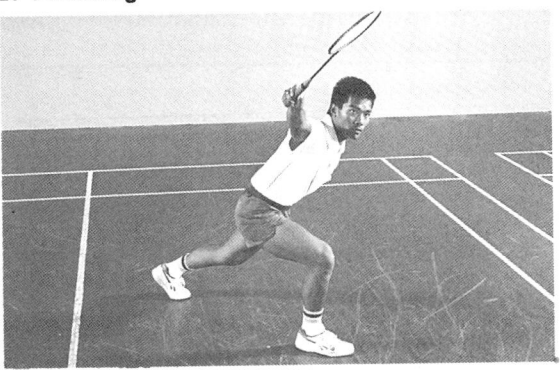

C. Contact

D. Follow-through

> ### Checklist for the Underhand Clear
>
> 1. Step to the shuttle with your right foot forward as you hit it.
> 2. Bring the racket head under the shuttle with your wrist cocked.
> 3. Hit hard, with a great deal of wrist action.
> 4. Follow through in your intended line of flight.

the shuttle. As you contact it, your forearm and wrist should whip your racket through the shuttle as you follow through in the intended direction of the flight of the shuttle. It should travel high and to the baseline area.

Underhand Drop

The underhand drop is played from behind the front service line. It is very similar to a low serve in that it should just clear the net, then drop quickly. This shot is valuable primarily in doubles play when played from midcourt. It can force a net player to move from side to side, or it can bring backcourt players to the net if they are playing side by side. In singles, it is generally used to return a smash, forcing the smashing player to cover some distance, then go on the defensive by hitting up.

Defensing the Smash

Defensing the smash is started by dropping your racket head low when you see that a smash is coming. It is best accomplished by *blocking* the smash crosscourt. (Your return may be a sidearm or an underhand stroke.)

The *block shot* is like the dab shot. It should land close to the net. Since it requires no backswing, you can use it to make the return even if you just barely get to the smash. If you don't have time to aim it, just block it straight. Your short shot will still give your opponent trouble.

A backhand shot gives you a greater range of blocking area—from shots aimed at the midline of your body to the non-racket sideline. With a forehand you have a range from in front of your racket-side leg to the sideline on your racket side.

Your return of the smash should get the shuttle back to an area that is difficult for your opponent to cover. Keep your opponent off-balance with a mix of drops, clears, and drives.

Also, smashes must be returned quickly; or the speed of the shuttle will have it past you in an instant.

The quickness required for your smash returns will limit you to primarily wrist shots. You won't have time to wind up and take a full backswing.

Keep your opponent guessing as to where you will return your shot.

In singles you will generally use a blocking action to return a smash,

Defensing a smash by dropping the racket head low

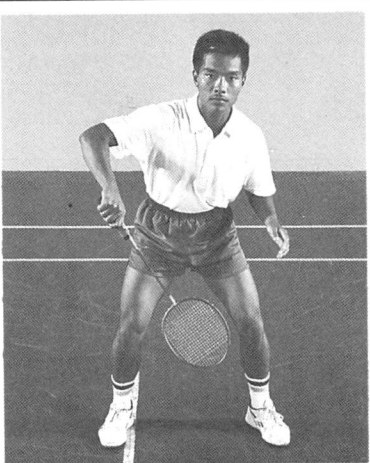

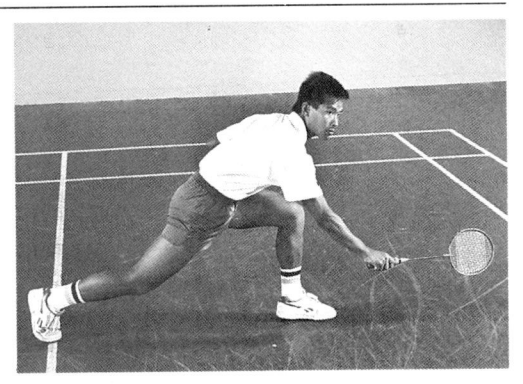

Backhand block of a smash

Blocking a smash at the body

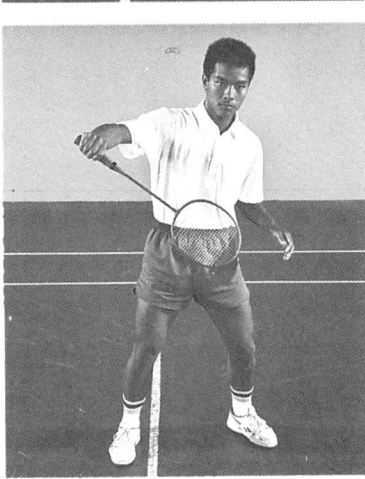

dropping the shuttle next to the net, an underhand drop, or a crosscourt block. In doubles you will generally use drive shots down the near sideline. For the blocks you simply get your racket in front of the shuttle and let the speed of the smashed shuttle provide part of the power for the return. For the drive shots you will have to supply some of the power needed with your wrist or arm.

On smashes aimed at the body, try to move your body away from the smash. It is easier to play a smash aimed at the backhand side of your body, because with the racket in your right hand, your hand will be farther from the shuttle. In any case, try to hit the shuttle as far in front of you as possible.

Hairpin Drop or Dribble

The *hairpin drop*, or *dribble*, is made close to the net after your opponent has hit a drop shot to you. The idea is to lift the shuttle gently over the top of the net and have it drop as close to the net as possible.

Hairpin drop:

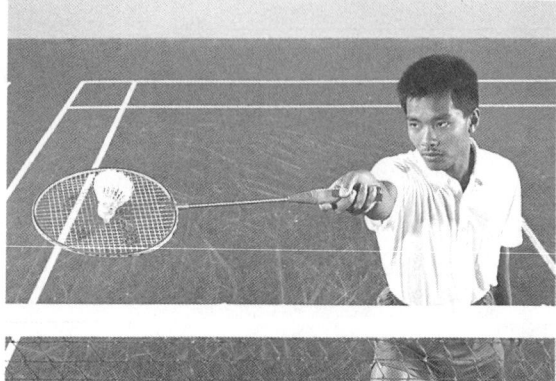

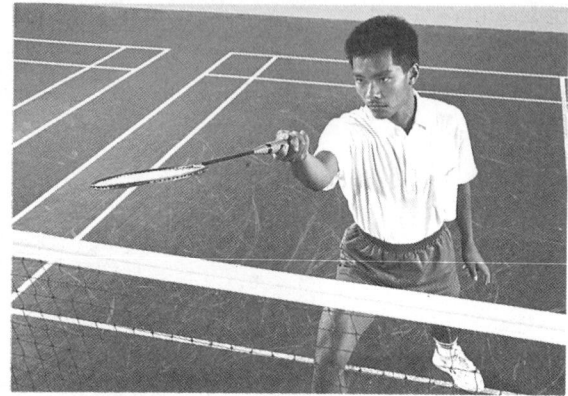

A. Contact

B. Follow-through

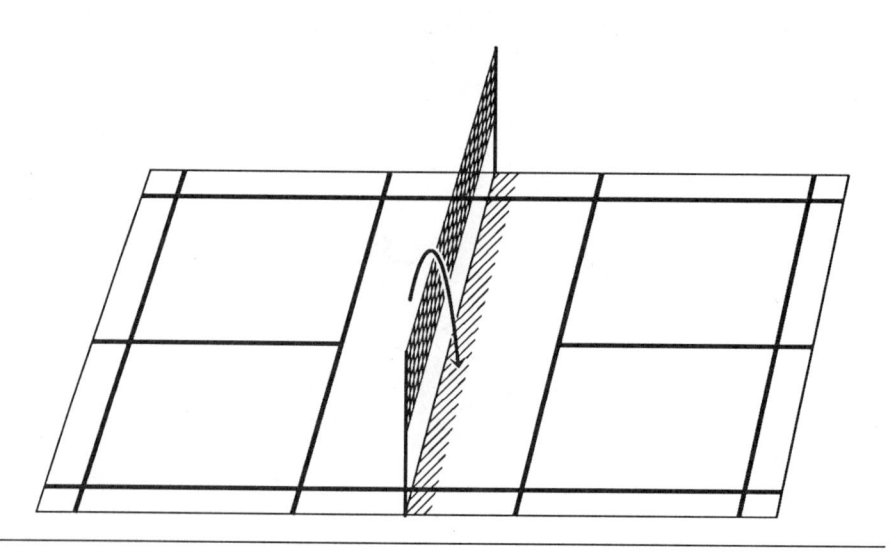

Get to the shuttle quickly, so that you can contact the shuttle as close to the top of the net as possible. In singles you don't have to be quite as precise with your placement as you do in doubles.

Your grip should be loose. Step toward the shuttle with your racket-side foot. The stroke is executed with your forearm and wrist. You should guide the shuttle over the net gently, and follow through with your forearm to give the desired direction.

You can place the shuttle directly in front of where you contact it, or you can guide it to a front corner of the court. Its flight path will be determined by the angle of your racket head at the point of contact.

Keep the shuttle close to the top of the net so that it cannot be smashed back at you. It should just clear the net and then drop. It is very difficult to return.

In doubles, with one person playing up and one back, you will be closer to the shuttle on this type of shot—but so is your opponent. You will have

> ### Checklist for the Hairpin Drop
>
> 1. Hold the racket loosely with a forehand grip.
> 2. Step with the right foot toward the shuttle.
> 3. Gently guide the shuttle over the net—as close to the top of the net as possible.

more area next to the net toward which to aim. You will need more variation and deception in your technique in order to hit safely to any spot in the forecourt. For that reason, when playing doubles you may want to *choke* up on your grip a bit (slide your hand up the handle) for better control.

Summary

1. While it is always preferable to hit with an overhead stroke, a good opponent will force you to hit many shots underhand.
2. Always try to use your underhand shot to get your opponent off-balance and to force a return to you that is high and short.
3. An effective drop shot at the net forces your opponent to hit the shuttle up. This may give you a set-up for a smash or a drive.
4. A high clear to your opponent can put him or her on the defensive.
5. One of the most effective shots to counter your opponent's drop shot is the dribble or hairpin drop.
6. On smash returns, block the shuttle as far in front of you as possible.

CHAPTER 8
Strategy

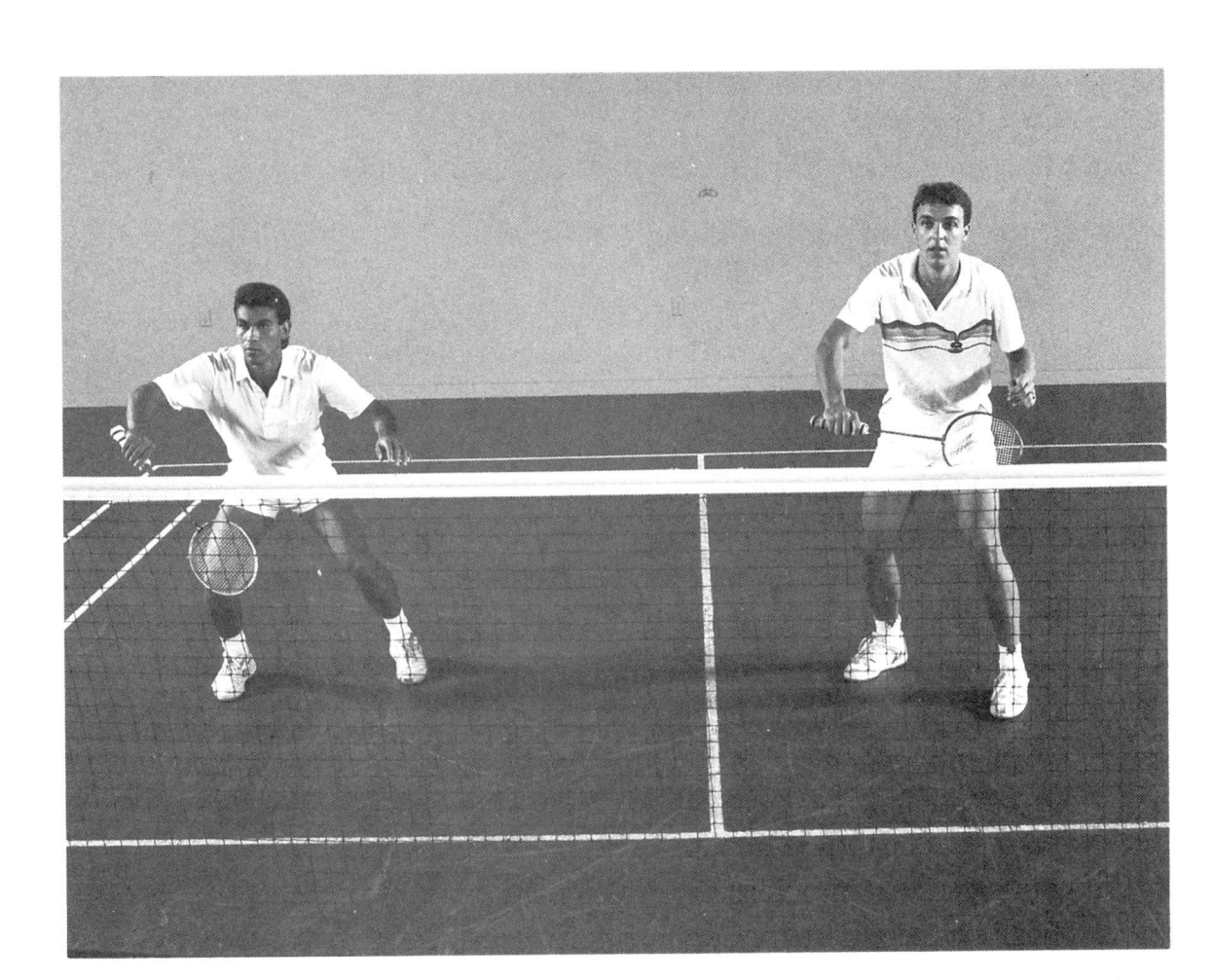

Outline

Basic Strategy
Your Fundamental Shots
Developing Game Strategy During Warm-Up
Singles Strategy
    Singles Serving
    Return of Service for Singles
    Singles Rally Strategy
Checklist for Singles Strategy
Doubles Strategy
    Doubles Serving
    Defensive Strategy for Doubles
    Offensive Strategy for Doubles
    Combination Strategy
Checklist for Doubles Strategy
Mixed Doubles Strategy
    Mixed Doubles Serving
    Return of Service for Mixed Doubles
    Mixed Doubles Play
Checklist for Mixed Doubles Strategy
Summary

One of the major thrills of badminton is outsmarting your opponent. Wise strategic decisions, if properly executed with good fundamentals, will win many games. As you gain experience and expertise, you will have more strategic options. In this chapter we will look at strategy from the beginning level to the more advanced levels.

Basic Strategy

1. Keep the shuttle away from your opponent.
2. Move your opponent out of the center of the court (the home-base position).
3. When in doubt, place the shuttle behind your opponent and hope for a weak return.
4. The backhand is usually the weaker side, so play to that.
5. While it is obvious that a left-hander's backhand is the same side as a right-hander's forehand, people often forget this. Remember to avoid hitting toward the forehand of a left-handed opponent under the mistaken notion that it is his or her backhand.
6. Return to your home-base position after every shot.
7. Use the smash to finish rallies, not as a basic shot to move your opponent and create openings.

Your Fundamental Shots

Good strategic decisions are wasted without good fundamentals. Remember these key points:

- Try always to hit the shuttle at as high a point as possible and as soon as possible. Don't wait for the shuttle to come to you. Move to it quickly and get behind it.
- Deception is a key element in this game, so you should attempt to make your strokes look similar as long as possible. For example, when a shot is hit high, you can fake a drop and hit a clear, or fake a smash and hit a drop.

Developing Game Strategy During Warm-Up

Try out various shots on your opponent during warm-up to see how he or she reacts to them. Especially try (1) drops to check your opponent's speed and ability and (2) clears to the backhand side to check on his or her strength there—and also to see if he or she runs around the backhand, thereby opening up an area to the forehand side.

Note whether your opponent seems slow or lazy. Is there a pattern to his or her returns, such as always hitting straight or crosscourt, or always clearing or dropping? Does your opponent want to smash too often, even when out of position or off-balance? These observations will help you plan your strategy.

If you are in a tournament, watch your future opponents in their matches to discover their strengths and weaknesses.

Target area for singles

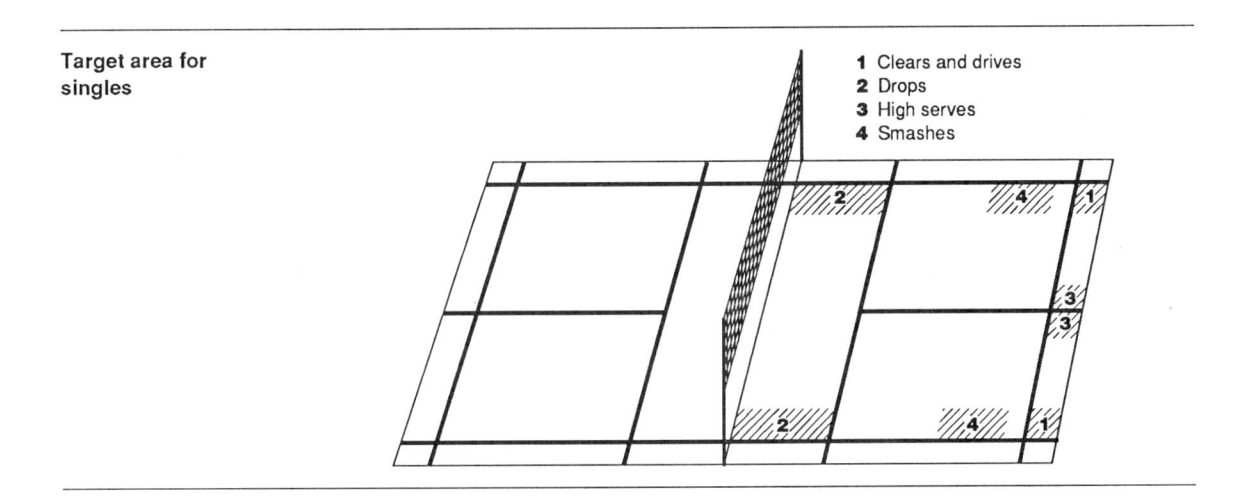

1 Clears and drives
2 Drops
3 High serves
4 Smashes

Singles Strategy

Most of your singles serves will be high and deep (whereas most of your doubles serves will be low and short). Throw in some flicks and drives, but mix them up so that your opponent cannot anticipate them. Try to be deceptive on your serves as well as on your strokes. And remember that if your serves are fast, the returns from your opponent are likely to be fast, so be ready for them.

Singles Serving

Singles serving is usually a high, deep shot to the back of the court near the midline. By serving near the midline of the backcourt, you cut down on the angle that your opponent can hit. But, again, vary your serves so that your opponent cannot guess exactly what you will do.

If your opponent is playing a bit too deep, hit a short serve. And if he or she is playing too close, hit the high, clear serve. Watch for evidence that one particular serve gives your opponent trouble.

Return of Service for Singles

Generally at the beginning level you will return both serves and shots straight ahead rather than placing them crosscourt, since the crosscourt shot takes longer and gives your opponent more time to adjust. Also, being a longer shot, it is more likely to fall shorter than intended and give your opponent an opening for a smash. But don't be predictable. You want to keep your opponent off-balance and guessing.

Your service return should move your opponent away from center court. The only time you would use a smash on a service return is on a high, short serve. Even then, use the smash only if you are certain that you can "put the bird on the floor." If you try to smash an effective serve, you will probably hit it weak, and you will be the one at a disadvantage.

The returns you'll use most often for a high serve are a high clear or a drop in the near corner away from your opponent. If a high serve is short (in front of the back doubles service line) you may smash, hit an attacking clear, or a drop to either near corner. If your opponent serves short and low, your best returns are a drop to the near corner or a flick or attacking clear, provided your opponent is close to the front service line.

Singles Rally Strategy

A primary rule of rally strategy is that whenever you get in trouble, you should hit the clear to your opponent's backhand. This gives you time to recover and may force your opponent into a weak return.

If you can get your opponent moving forward and back you will have an advantage. Try to move him or her into the various corners of the court and away from the controlling position in the center of the court. By moving your opponent, you may force weak returns and create holes in his or her defense. For you to keep control of the rally, you must maintain your strong position at your home base.

A popular combination is a clear to the backhand, then a drop to the forehand, followed by another deep backhand clear and another forehand drop. This makes your opponent move a great distance and execute a weak shot (the high backhand) at the end of a long run.

With a continued pattern of clears and drops, you will eventually force your opponent to hit a weak return. This is the time for you to win the point with a smash. You must have both patience and endurance for this defensive type of strategy. Once you get your opponent moving, you can take the offensive. Vary your shots. You can hit a hard drive or a smash directly at your opponent as he or she charges the net. If your opponent runs quickly forward after you have hit a clear, you might hit two clears in a row. You can then hit a drive behind your opponent as he or she is moving in the opposite direction.

While every player should be adept at both offensive shots and defensive shots, before starting serious training you should determine whether you want to emphasize the offensive or defensive aspects of your game. Which style fits you best?

Checklist for Singles Strategy

1. Move your opponent from the home-base position to the corners.
2. Force your opponent to hit up (play defensively) as often as possible.
3. Hit deep, especially to the backhand, to force weak returns.
4. Hit the shuttle as early and as high as possible.
5. Disguise your shots and vary them.
6. When returning smashes, hit deep or short—never to the midcourt area.

Block, straight, smash cross-court

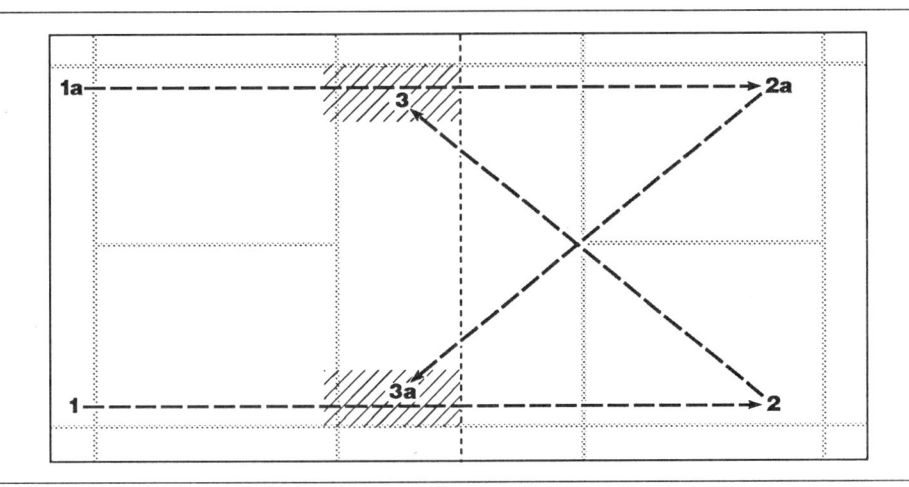

If you are strong and can hit hard, you may opt to be an attacking player. If you are quick, have stamina, and perhaps are shorter than average, you might choose to play a more defensive game. In either case you will need to practice all of your fundamentals, because the offensive players will use many clears and drops, and the defensive players will sometimes use the smash.

To defend a smash, block it, and drop it close to the net. If your opponent has smashed straight, you might drop it crosscourt. If your opponent has smashed crosscourt, drop it in the near front corner.

If you are trailing your opponent's score late in a game, you might switch your strategy to a safer one called the *center court theory,* in which you avoid the sidelines in your shots. Hit smashes at your opponent's body—between the waist and shoulder of the racket side of the body. Such a strategy reduces your chance of hitting the shuttle out of bounds, and it reduces the angle of return by your opponent. (Note: This is an exception to the badminton courtesy of avoiding hits into the body of an opponent as a common practice.)

Block, cross-court, smash, straight

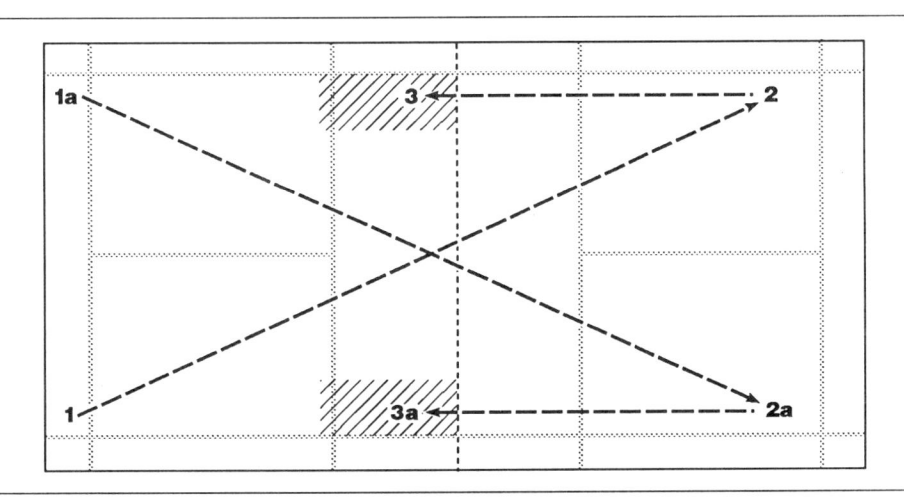

Doubles Strategy

Doubles is a more complex game than singles. It demands faster reactions and being able to anticipate what your partner and your opponents will do with the shuttle. Good doubles play begins with an effective serve or service return (the most important parts of the game) and ends with good teamwork on offense.

Doubles Serving

The server in a doubles game must vary the placement of the serve in order to prevent the opponent from attacking the serve. The short serve, the drive, and the high flick serves are used in doubles. The low, short serve to the near corner (the diagonal "T" area) is the most common serve. Top-caliber servers can often make points with a shot that is generally thought to be defensive.

Deception, an essential in the game of badminton, is particularly important in the serve. Make certain that the beginning of your serving action is the same for every type of serve you execute.

Return of Service for Doubles

The return for beginners should start with the ready position taken a few feet back from the front service line. As you become advanced, you will move up to within one foot of the front service line and within one foot of the centerline. From this point any low serves can be played quickly and at a high point.

Drop returns should be played straight ahead, not crosscourt. Drive returns should be at the backhand or down the near sideline. Push returns should be at the near sideline and to midcourt.

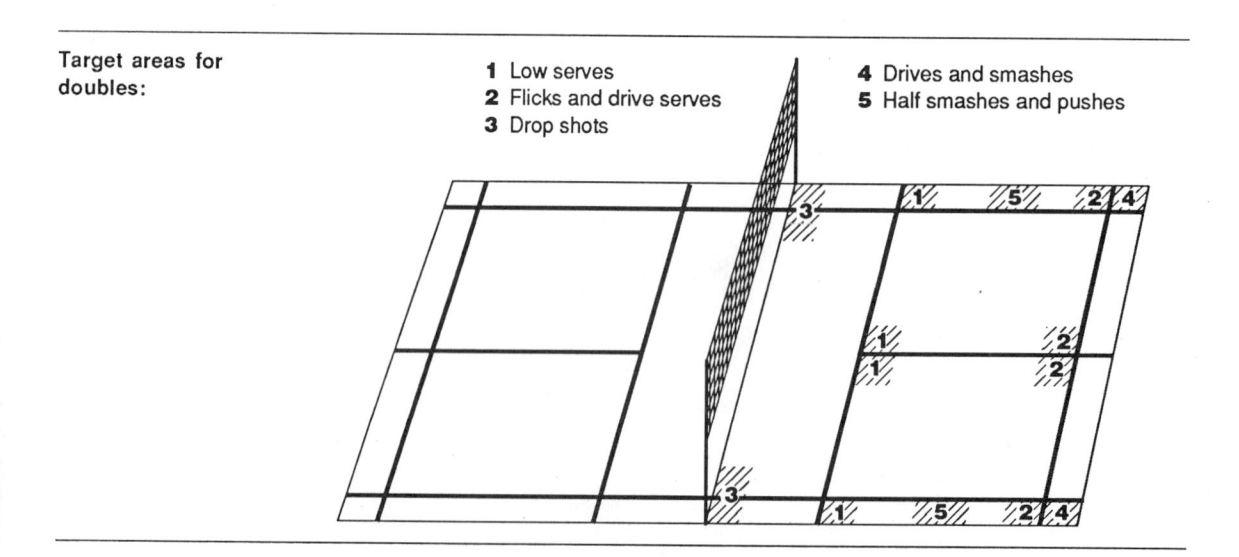

Target areas for doubles:
1 Low serves
2 Flicks and drive serves
3 Drop shots
4 Drives and smashes
5 Half smashes and pushes

Target areas for doubles return

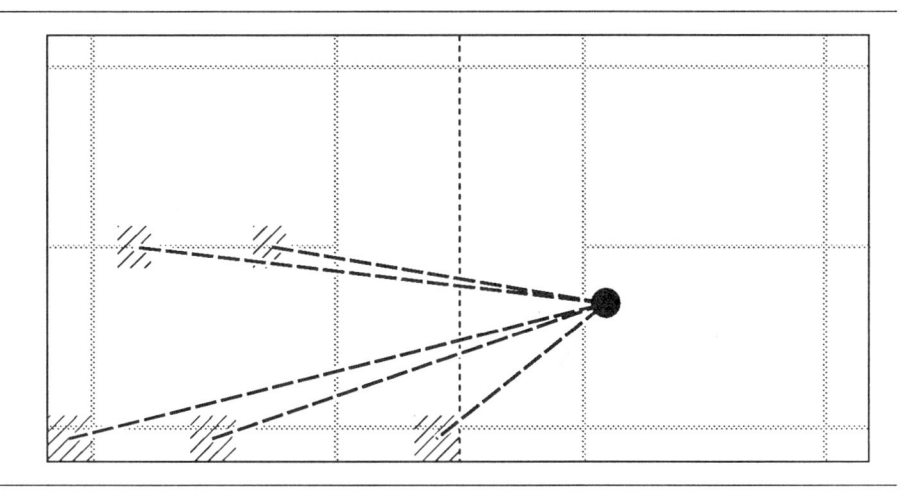

The best service returns for doubles are

- A push along the near sideline to midcourt.
- A drop shot away from the server's side.
- A drive to the deep corner on the near side.
- A push shot just behind the server.
- A push into the body of the server's partner.

Defensive Strategy for Doubles
Effective service, service return, and rallies in doubles play all begin with proper alignment. Start your play from the best position for what you want to accomplish. You can play a defensive alignment (*side by side*), an offensive alignment (*up and back*), or you can use a combination of these two formations, called *circular rotation*, depending on the situation in the game.

Side-by-side alignment for doubles

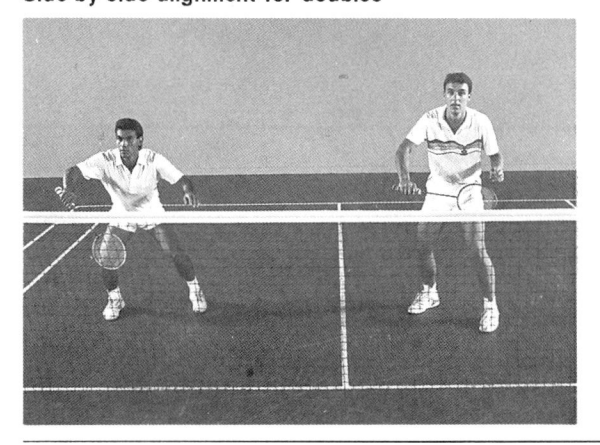

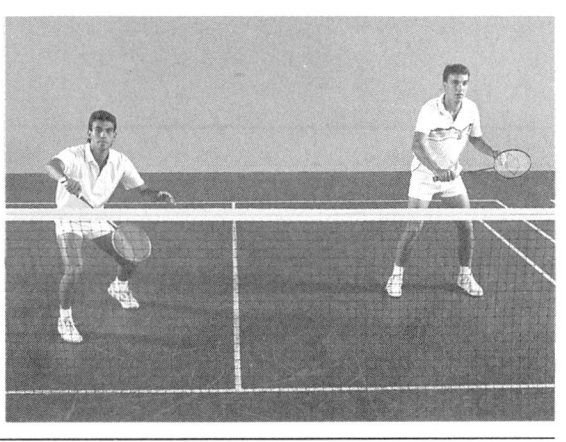

BADMINTON TODAY

Basic side-by-side doubles alignment, with each player responsible for his or her half-court

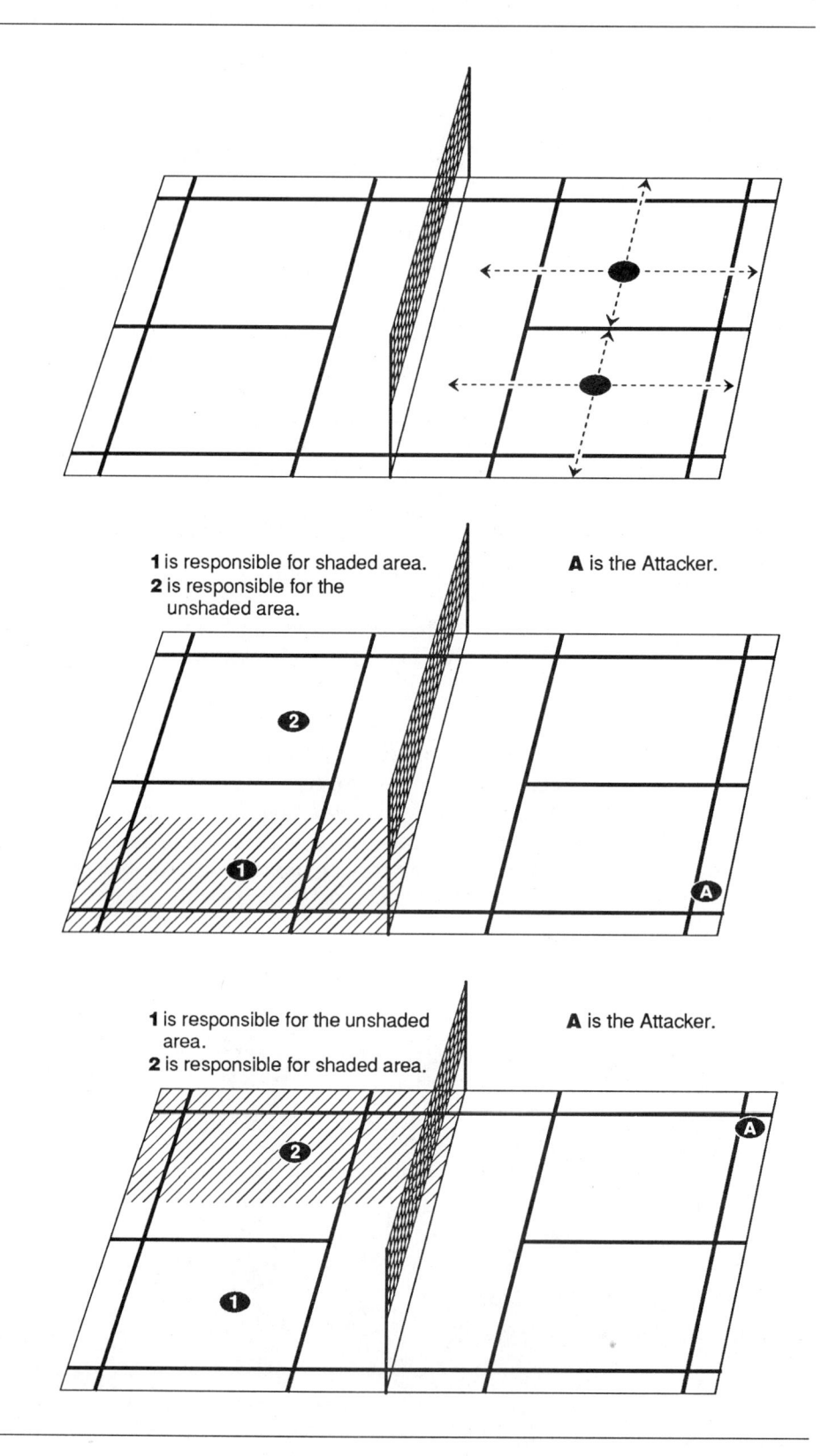

1 is responsible for shaded area.
2 is responsible for the unshaded area.

A is the Attacker.

1 is responsible for the unshaded area.
2 is responsible for shaded area.

A is the Attacker.

In the *side-by-side alignment*, the basic defensive position for doubles, each partner is responsible for his or her half of the court. This alignment is easy to learn and eliminates confusion as to who will take a shot.

The defender directly in front of the attacker takes all shuttles that are hit to the sideline, all drop shots to his or her side of the court, all shots at the body, and all the high clears down the middle. The partner, who turns slightly toward the attacker, takes all the smashes hit to the center of the court or crosscourt and all drop shots on his or her side of the court.

This side-by-side alignment makes it much more difficult for your opponents to smash effectively. A drawback, however, is that it allows your opponents to continue to play to the weaker partner, not only obtaining weaker returns but also tiring him or her. Also, as a defensive rather than an offensive formation, it reduces a team's chance to attack, and doubles is an offensive game.

To get back on offense, a team using this alignment should block or push its opponents' smashes into the halfcourt area or clear them crosscourt. The attacker should be forced to run sideways to maintain his or her attack. This way he or she will not be able to hit deep, angled smashes, and hence the defenders will have a better chance of playing halfcourt returns and getting back on offense.

Side-by-side alignment is the best strategy when your opponents are in control. However, it should be remembered that attacking (offensive strategy) rather than defending is generally the best plan for winning at doubles.

Offensive Strategy for Doubles

The *up-and-back alignment* for offensive play places both players in the midline of the court with one player close to the net, about one foot behind the "T" (the intersection of the midline and the short service line) and the other playing deep. This alignment (also easy to learn) is more effective against a team that hits strong, deep clears and short drops. One of its advantages is that the weaker player can be "hidden" at the net, with the stronger player playing most of the court. Another is that it is an attacking formation. Disadvantages are

Up-and-back alignment for doubles

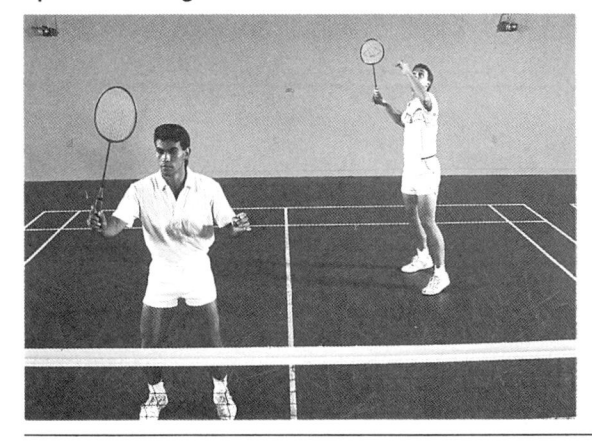

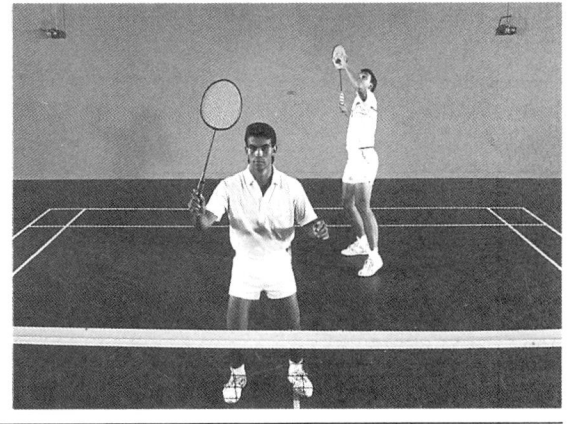

that the sides of the court are open to the smash and your opponents can run the backcourt player from side to side to tire him or her.

The normal pattern is for the server to play the "up" position after serving. The person receiving will play up if the serve is short and will play deep if the serve is long—with the partner playing the opposite position. In more advanced doubles the stronger person will generally play deep and the weaker person up.

Both players must keep the shuttle low to the opponents. Any time that the shuttle is hit high the net player becomes a sitting duck for a smash.

When playing the up-and-back alignment, if you are the up player do not turn and look toward your partner. Keep your eyes on your opponents. There are two reasons for this. One is that you can get hit in the face with your partner's shot. The other is that by watching your opponents, you will know where the shuttle is going and will be able to adjust to its return more quickly.

The deeper player should adjust his or her position by playing slightly to the other side of the court from the up person. So if the up player is forced to the right, the back player will move to the left.

The success of offensive doubles depends to a large degree on the person playing near the net. This player can block shots and drop them close to the net—forcing the opponents into weak returns. Most rallies in good doubles are won by the net player.

The net player should take a position one and one-half to two feet ahead of the short service line. The racket should be held near net level. From this position you can move side to side and cut off most short shots. On a smash the forecourt player should defend the opposite side of the court from where the attacker is. This means that the forecourt player moves away from the centerline and back behind the short service line (see diagram).

From this position the forecourt player should be able to make downward shots that the attackers will have to pop up. If it is not possible to hit the shuttle down, it should be blocked near the net to keep the opponents on the defensive.

The backcourt player should attempt to hit smashes down the line, into the center of the court, or into the body of the opponent who is nearest. The speed and angle of the smash should be varied to keep the opponents off-balance. Power is not as important in winning at doubles as variety and consistency.

Partners should be able to adjust to each other and to the expected shots of their opponents. For example, if the net player has hit a drop shot, the backcourt player can move up, expecting that the opponents will counter with another drop shot.

Experienced players will be able to see if their opponents have moved forward or are too far back. They can then adjust their shots to take advantage of the resulting openings. Players who have played together for a long time will learn their partners' strengths and weaknesses and be able to set up their partners so that they make strong shots.

Combination Strategy

Combination of the side-by-side and up-and-back strategies is possible for more advanced players. As you get to know your partner, you can switch between

Up-and-back doubles alignment and court responsibilities

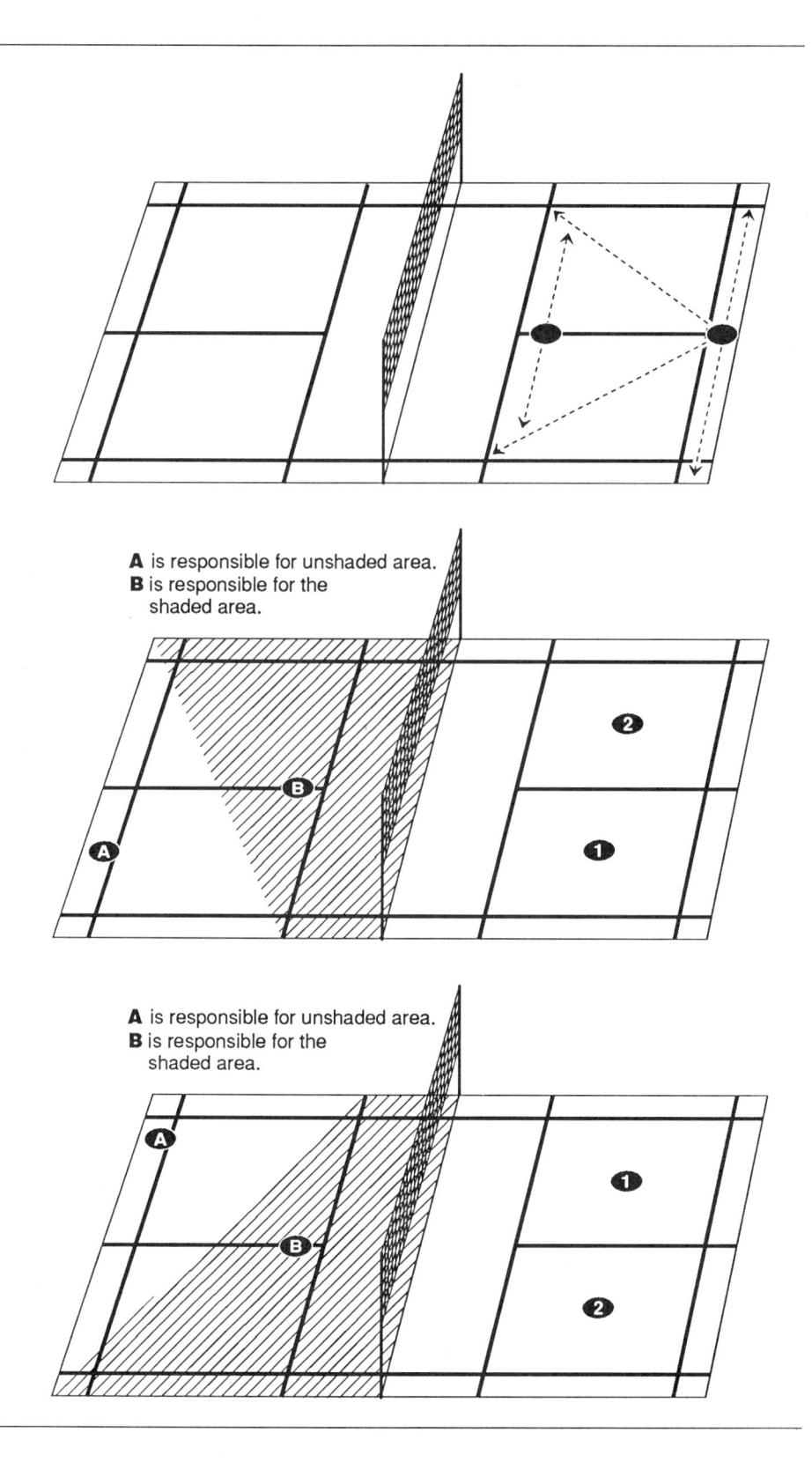

A is responsible for unshaded area.
B is responsible for the shaded area.

A is responsible for unshaded area.
B is responsible for the shaded area.

> **Checklist for Doubles Strategy**
>
> 1. Against an up-and-back team
>   a. Play to the weaker opponent.
>   b. Hit shots to the corners to make opponents move up and back.
> 2. Against a side-by-side team
>   a. Hit midcourt level shots to the sidelines.
>   b. Hit shots to the corners to make opponents move sideways and to hit weaker returns or hit up.
>   c. Smash to the sidelines as often as possible.

side-by-side and up-and back- formations. Usually, if you hit the shuttle down, as in a drop, smash, or drive, you will go on offense and play up and back. If you lift the shuttle, you will likely go on defense and play side-by-side. A lower-level player may use verbal signals to alert the partner to a change, but advanced players learn to react to the proper position depending on the shot.

Mixed Doubles Strategy

At the championship level men are generally stronger, taller, and faster than women. In physical education classes these differences may not exist. For this reason mixed doubles strategy will be discussed in terms of the stronger and weaker player rather than the man and the woman.

Mixed Doubles Serving

The basic serve in mixed doubles is the short serve. However, doubles players should also have an effective flick serve in order to be able to take advantage of any weaknesses in the opponents' alignment or fundamental skills.

The short serve is usually served to the "T" (the intersection of the front service line with the midline.) A wide short serve to the side of the court is usually not employed because the *down-the-line* return of serve is simple to execute and difficult to defend against.

A flick serve can be used more often against the shorter and weaker (and therefore probably slower) player, from the usual position at the net. It may also create gaps in the defense and allow the serving team to "put the bird on the floor."

The weaker player, who will be covering the shots close to the net, will serve from close to the front service line. The stronger player may serve from deeper in order to be ready for a high, clear return.

Return of Service for Mixed Doubles

The return of service is very important in mixed doubles. If the serve is poor (i.e., too high at the net) the receiver should move quickly to hit the shuttle down. The best return is usually straight back into the server at waist level and into the racket side of the body.

If the stronger player serves short and tight to the weaker opponent, the returner can make a net return to the sideline. A crosscourt net return might be intercepted by the opposing net player. Other times the shuttle can be pushed into the deep corners of the court before the stronger player is able to get back to cover them.

If the weaker player is serving to the weaker player on the other team, the returns should be straight ahead or dropped into the corner away from the server. Any crosscourt returns can be intercepted by the server and dabbed to the floor.

Short returns to the outside corners should be returned straight, regardless of who is serving.

In high-level competition, when the stronger player returns a serve from the weaker opponent, the shuttle should be pushed into the face or body of the weaker opponent. Another effective return is the halfcourt push to the sidelines. Avoid making a net shot straight ahead, because it can be cleared quickly over the stronger player's head, forcing the weaker partner to go into the backcourt.

When the stronger player returns service from an opposing strong player, the shuttle should be pushed to the sidelines at about halfcourt depth. It is most important for the stronger player to hit the return downward. After the return, the stronger player should move quickly to the backcourt to protect that area. The strongest alignment in mixed doubles is to have the weaker player up and the stronger player back. This puts the team in the best offensive position.

When either partner receives a flick serve, it should be smashed to the sidelines or into the server's body. Once in a while a fast drop or half-smash at the alley can be attempted.

Mixed Doubles Play

The play in mixed doubles should be concentrated toward the sidelines because the partners will be generally playing up and back. The shuttle should be hit down to make the opponents hit upward. If you are forced to hit a high, clear shot, move into a *wedge formation*, because your opponents will probably hit a smash. In the wedge formation the stronger player aligns in front of the smasher and fairly deep in the court. The responsibility is for all shots to that side of the court. The weaker player defends the other side of the court and aligns shorter to take crosscourt and midcourt shots and drops. The racket should be held in front of the body with the head of the racket at head height.

Try to move the net player, usually the weaker player, from side to side with fast drops and crosscourt net shots. The shuttle should be played flat and directed down the sidelines. Crosscourt flat shots can be easily cut off by the opposing net player. However, if the deep player wants to hit a crosscourt

Wedge formation

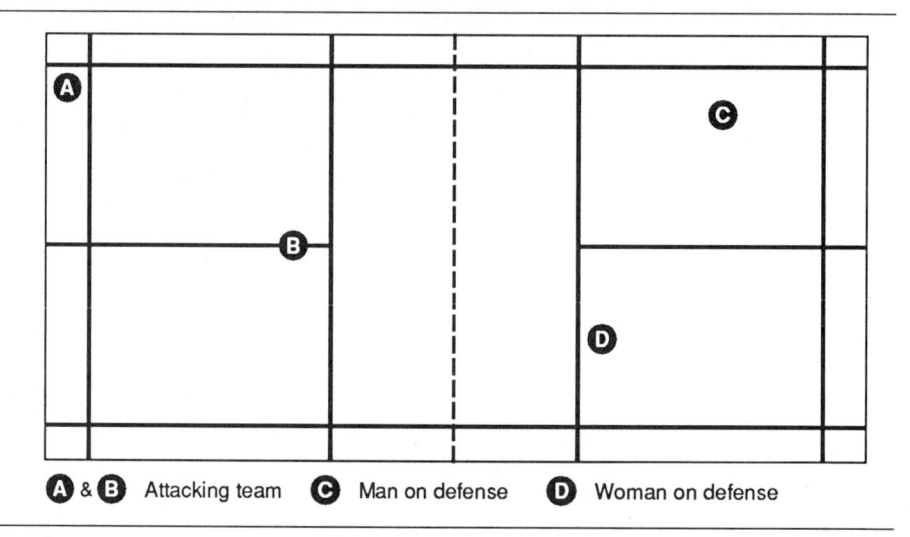

A & **B** Attacking team   **C** Man on defense   **D** Woman on defense

shot, it should be hit over the head of the opposing net player to push him or her into the backcourt.

The net player, in general, should not try to intercept the straight halfcourt pushes unless he or she is certain of a good return. The net player should be content playing a good net game by hitting low net shots—not by hitting clears. When the shuttle is returned a bit higher than the top of the net, it should be smashed. The net player should hit every shot down, whether it be a drop, a drive, or a push.

On defense a wedge formation can be used when you have hit a high, weak return and expect a smash. The weaker player moves back a few steps and takes a position to intercept crosscourt smashes and drops. The smashes should be blocked away from the opposing net player.

Checklist for Mixed Doubles Strategy

1. Play to the near sidelines.
2. Move the net player from side to side.
3. Try to hit every shot down.
4. Most serves should be low.

Summary

1. Simple strategy includes
   a. Keeping the shuttle away from your opponent.
   b. Moving your opponent from the home-base position.
   c. When in doubt, hitting a high clear to your opponent's backhand.
2. Singles serving strategy is based on serving mostly high deep serves.
3. Singles strategy is designed to keep your opponent away from the home-base position.
4. The smash is the most overused stroke in badminton.
5. Doubles is a more complex game than singles.
6. The serve is the most important part of a doubles game. Serves should be short and low or higher flick serves. Keep your opponent off-balance.
7. The side-by-side alignment is a defensive formation.
8. The up-and-back alignment is an offensive formation.

CHAPTER 9

Drills

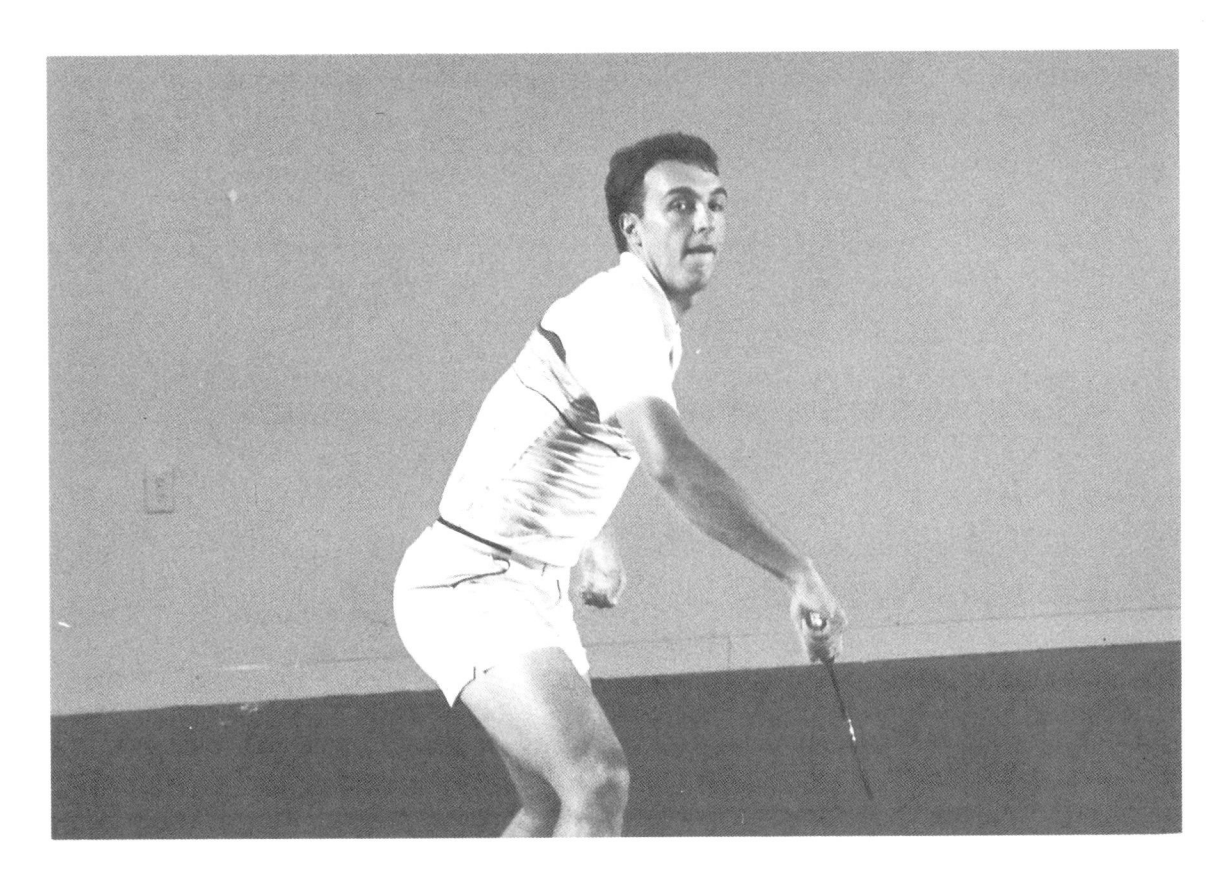

Outline

Drills
1. Serving Drills
2. High Service Return Drills
3. Low Service Return Drills
4. Straight Clear
5. Crosscourt Clear
6. Combination Down-the-Line and Crosscourt Drills
7. Overhead Clear-and-Drop Combination
8. Smash Drill
9. Smash-and-Block Drill
10. Smash-and-Halfcourt Drive
11. Drives
12. Drops
13. Alternating Drops
14. Overhead Drop and Underhand Clear
15. Net Shots (Hairpin Drops and Cross-Net Shots)
16. Quickness Drill
17. Clear, Smash, Drop, Clear
18. Doubles Drill

Self-Tests
1. Deep Singles Serves
2. Low Doubles Serve
3. Forehand and Backhand Clears
4. Drop Shots
5. Smash

Summary

Drills

In any sport the best players are the ones who work the most on their fundamental skills. Badminton is no exception. The more you practice, the more you will improve your game. Here are some drills to incorporate into your practice sessions.

1. Serving Drills
This drill can be done with or without a partner. The server simply hits the desired serve, high clear, short, flick, or drive), and the partner—if there is one—lets the shuttle drop to see how close to the desired corner it lands. When doing this drill alone, use several shuttles.

2. High Service Return Drills
A partner is required to serve a high clear. It is returned with the smash, clear, or drop.

3. Low Service Return Drills
A partner is required to serve a low serve to either front corner of the doubles court. Taking the proper alignment near the front service line, and close to the centerline, you return the serve with the underhand clear, drive, push, drop, or rushing-net shot.

4. Straight Clear
Partners hit to each other, from the backcourt then from the forecourt, attempting to get the shuttle to drop straight down within one foot of the backline. Every so often, a player can let the shuttle drop to see just how close it was to the baseline.

5. Crosscourt Clear
Players both hit crosscourt clears, working for distance and placement into the corner box—the area between the singles and doubles sidelines and the

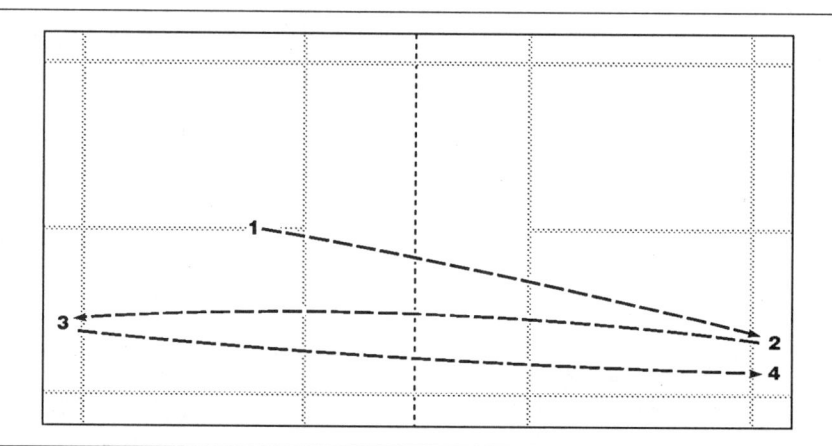

Straight clear (4)

Crosscourt clear (6)

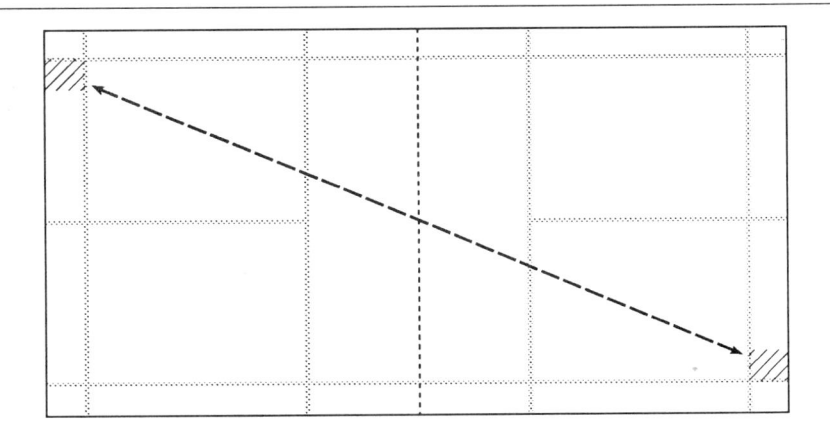

deep doubles service line and the baseline. This drill should be done forehand to forehand or, for advanced players, backhand to backhand.

6. Combination Down-the-Line and Crosscourt Clears

1. Players start in home-base position and hit down-the-line clears, returning to home base after each shot.
2. Players start in home-base position and hit crosscourt clears, returning to home base after each shot.
3. Players alternate between down-the-line and crosscourt shots, returning to home base after each shot.

7. Overhead Clear-and-Drop Combination

One player hits all clears while the other alternates between hitting an overhead clear and a drop. Emphasis with the advanced players should be to disguise the shots so that the windup of the backswing and the forward swing look similar.

Overhead clear-and-drop combination (7)

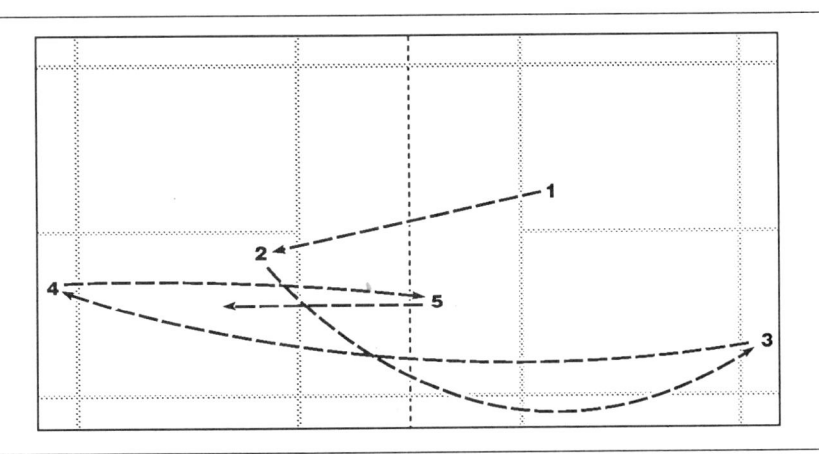

Smash drill (8)

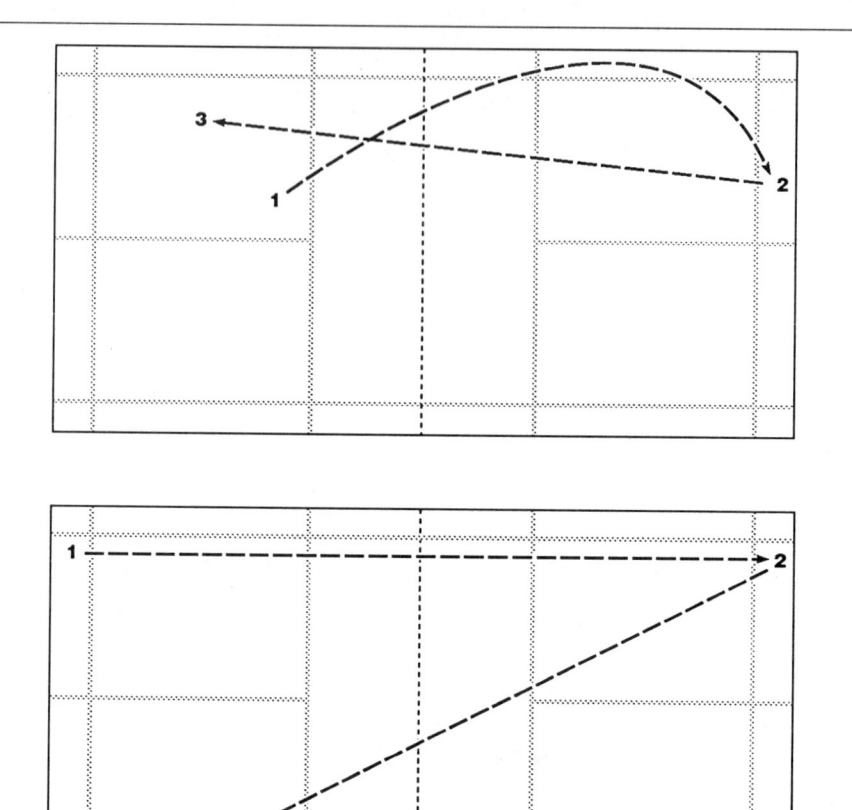

8. Smash Drill
One player hits short, high clears while the other smashes.

9. Smash-and-Block Drill
One player hits a short, high clears, which the partner smashes. The returner attempts to block the smash straight ahead.

10. Smash-and-Halfcourt Drive
Similar to the smash-and block drill, but the returner applies more power to the return and hits a halfcourt drive.

11. Drives
Each player hits drive drives to each other down the near sideline. One player's forehand shot will be played by the other's backhand.

DRILLS 93

Smash-and-block drill (9)

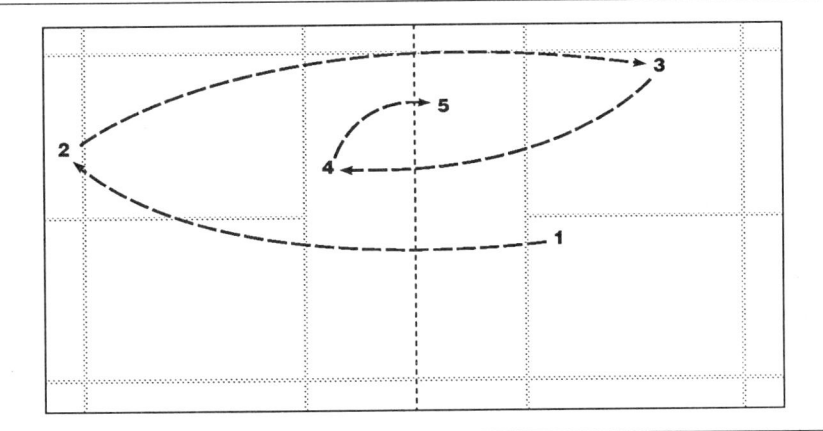

Smash-and-block drive (10)

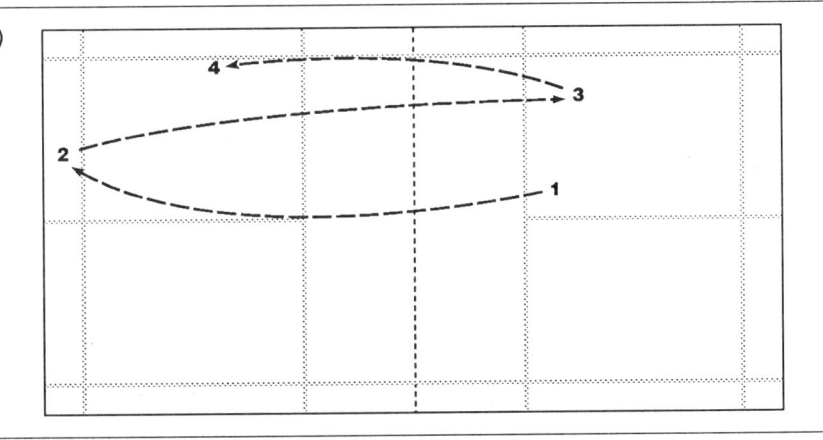

Drives (11)

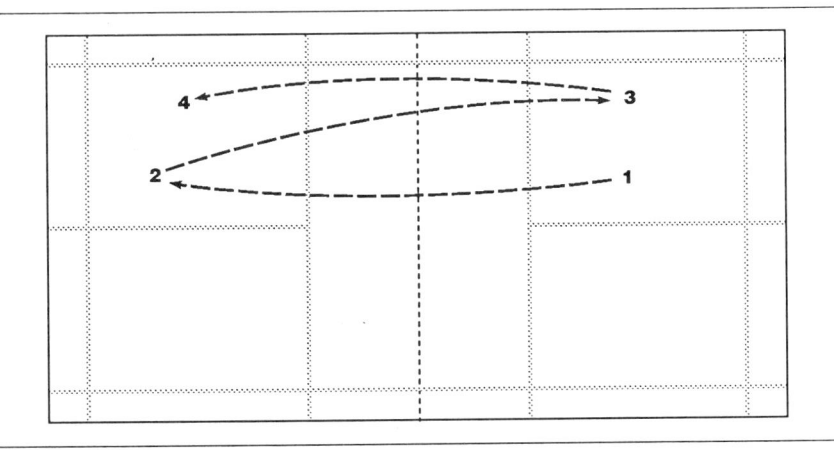

Drops (12)

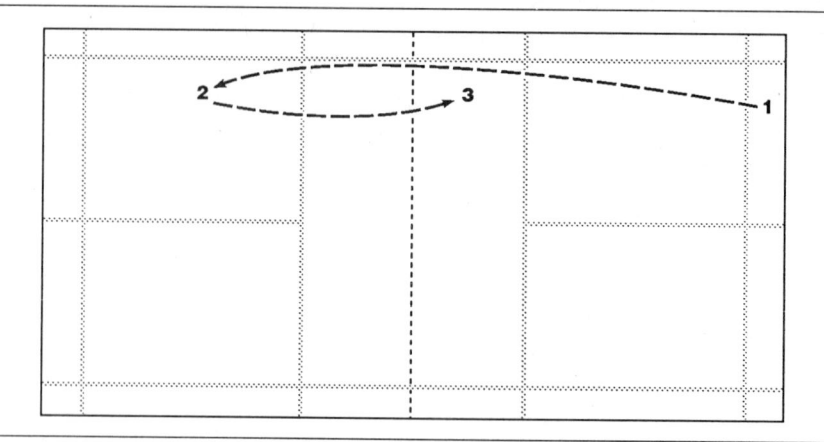

Alternating Drops (13)

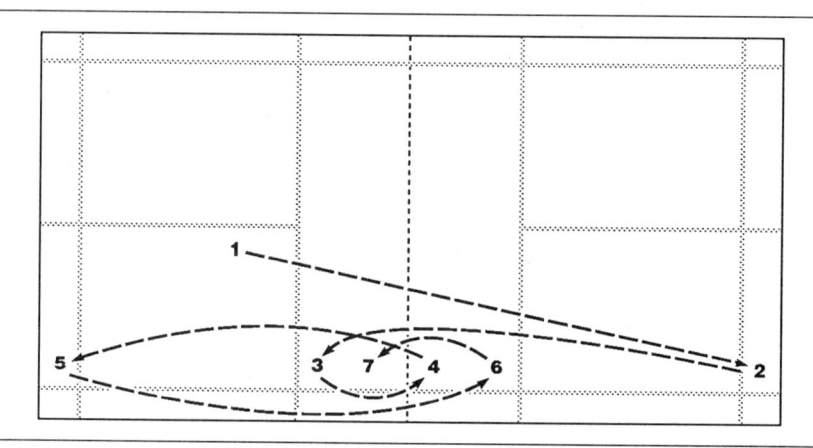

12. Drops
Partners hit drops, straight and crosscourt, to each other straight ahead. They then work on the crosscourt drop. The shuttle should just clear the net on each shot.

13. Alternating Drops
Both persons hit drops alternately.

14. Overhead Drop and Underhand Clear
One player hits only drops, while the partner hits only clears.

15. Net Shots (Hairpin Drops and Cross-Net Shots)
Players practice hairpin drops, then crosscourt net shots, then hit them in combination—trying to score on the other net player.

16. Quickness Drill
Players stand on the "T" and hit drive shots at and to each other. One can hit all forehands while the other hits all backhands. They can then rally as quickly as possible, hitting all drives (no clears or drops). By hitting some drives at each other, they can learn how to defend against this type of shot. This drill helps the player learn how to watch the shuttle and react quickly.

Overhead drop and underhand clear (14)

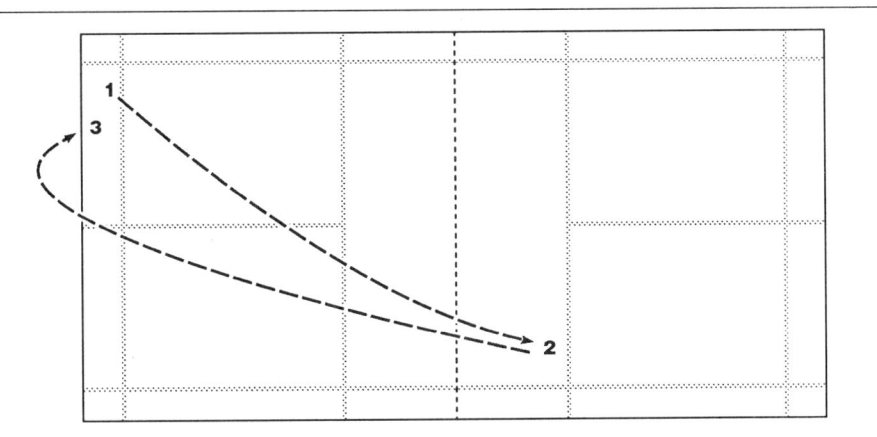

Net shots: Hairpin drops (15)

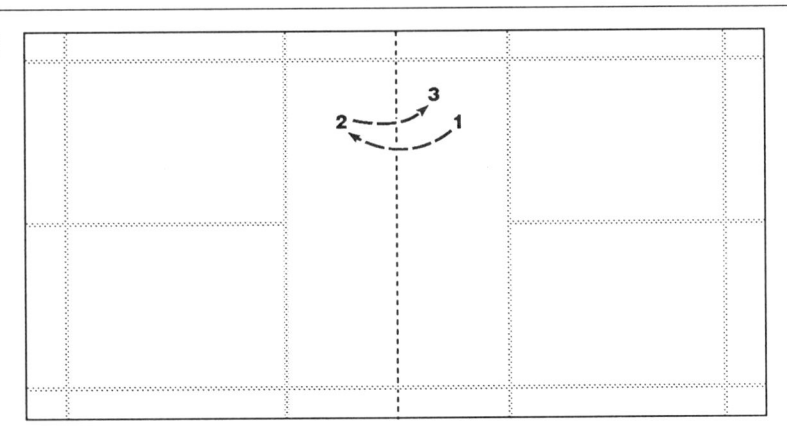

Cross-net shot (15)

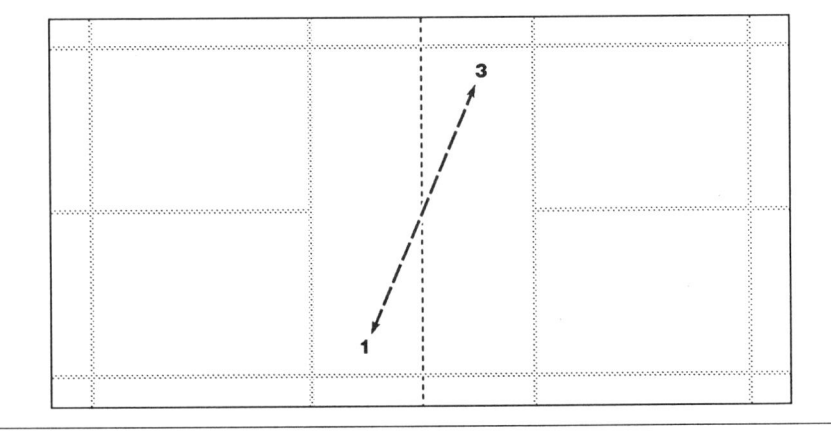

Clear, smash, drop, clear (17)

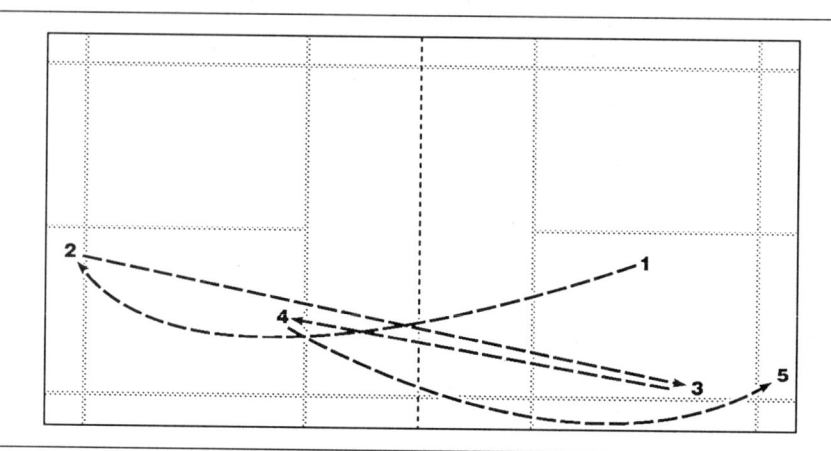

Doubles drill (18)

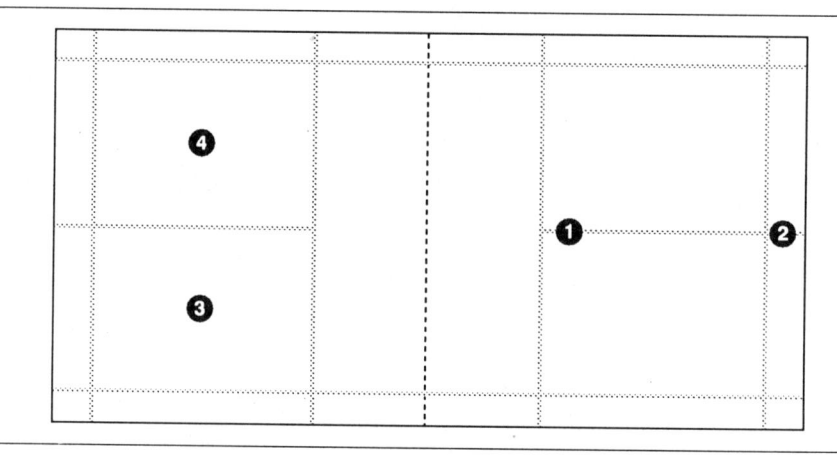

17. Clear, Smash, Drop, Clear
One player hits a clear, the partner returns it with a smash, the smash is returned with a drop, and the drop is returned with a clear. The cycle is repeated. The order of shots for the first player is clear, drop, smash, clear, drop, smash, etc. For the second player, it is smash, clear, drop, smash, clear, drop, etc. In other words, partners smash the clear, drop-shot the smash, and clear the drop shot. This pattern is continued until one person misses, then it is started again.

18. Doubles Drill
One team plays defensively, in side-by-side formation, and the other offensively, in up-and-back formation. All of the doubles skills can be practiced in this drill.

Self-Tests

Self-tests may be made more complex depending on skill level (i.e. adding specific targets). The following are directed to beginners.

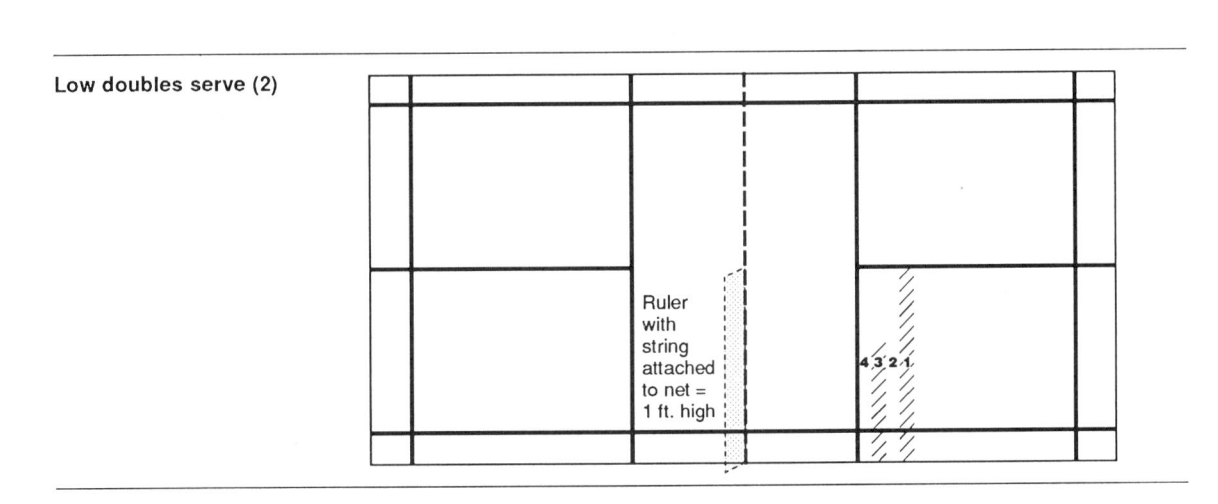

1. Deep Singles Serves
Mark the court from the baseline forward in 2-foot increments. Take ten serves. If you serve the shuttle into the deepest section, give yourself 4 points. The next section in is worth 3 points, the next section 2 points, and the closest section is 1 point. A perfect score would be 40 points.

2. Low Doubles Serve
Mark the court in 1-foot increments from the service line back. Take ten serves. If you serve low (within 1 foot of the net) and to the closest area (short service line to 1 foot back), give yourself 4 points. The next area (1 foot to 2 feet from the service line) is worth 3, the next area (2 to 3 feet from the short service line) is worth 2 points, and the farthest area (3 to 4 feet from the service line) is worth 1. A perfect score would be 40 points.

3. Forehand and Backhand Clears
Mark the court with four 2-feet increments starting from the backline. From a position in the backcourt, a partner will hit you ten shots to your forehand

Forehand and backhand clears (3)

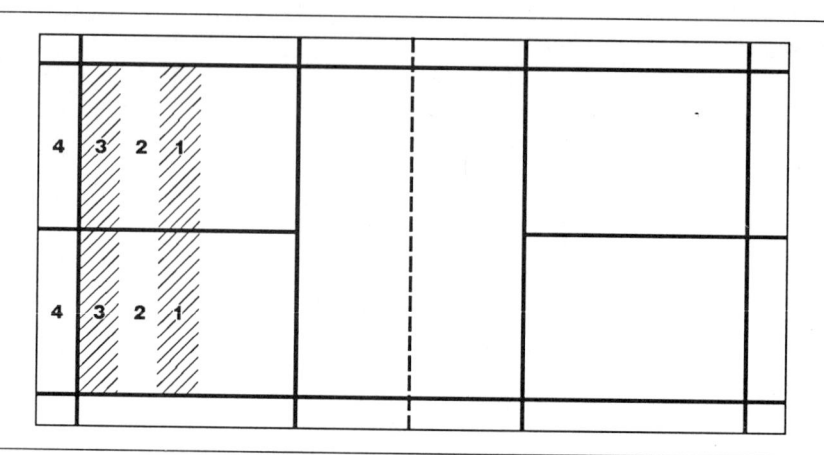

Drop shots (4)

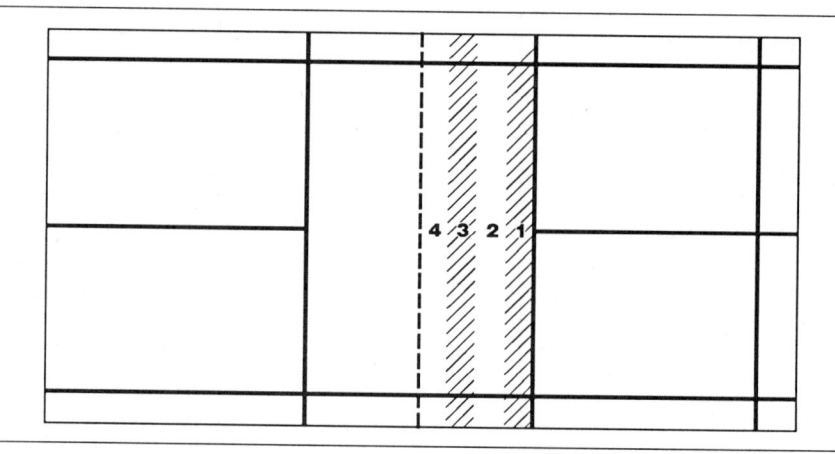

and then ten to your backhand. Your scores will be 1, 2, 3, or 4 depending on which increment area you hit your high clear shot into. From the end line to 2 feet in is 4 points, from 2 to 4 feet in is 3 points, etc.

(Note: a more advanced player may be needed to "feed" the shuttle into the backcourt.)

4. Drop Shots
With the court marked in 2-foot increments from the net, and you playing from near the midcourt, hit ten drop shots. The score is 4 if the shuttle lands within 2 feet of the net, 3 if it lands 2 to 4 feet from the net, 3 if it lands 2 feet inside the service line, and 4 if it lands 2 feet past the service line.

5. Smash
While standing midcourt, have a partner set you up with a short clear. Smash into the other court. You get 4 points if you hit the shuttle between the back

Smash (5)

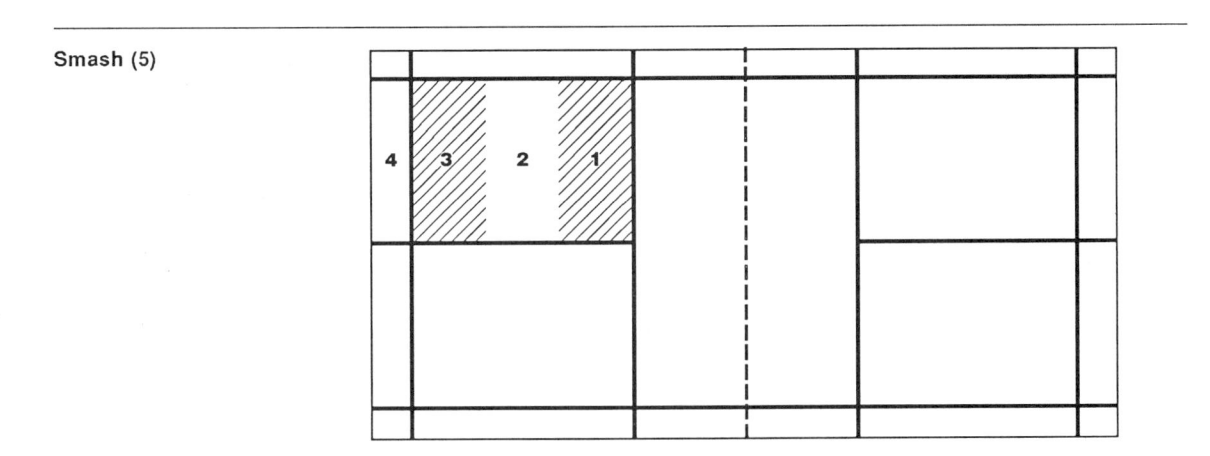

boundary line and the back doubles service court line, 3 points if you hit it from the back doubles court line to a point 4 feet forward of that point, 2 points if you hit it from the next closest 4-foot area, and 1 point if you hit it from the service line to 4 feet back.

Summary

1. Drills are essential to making rapid progress in any sport.
2. Concentrate on what you are doing.

CHAPTER 10

Increasing Your Mental and Physical Potentials

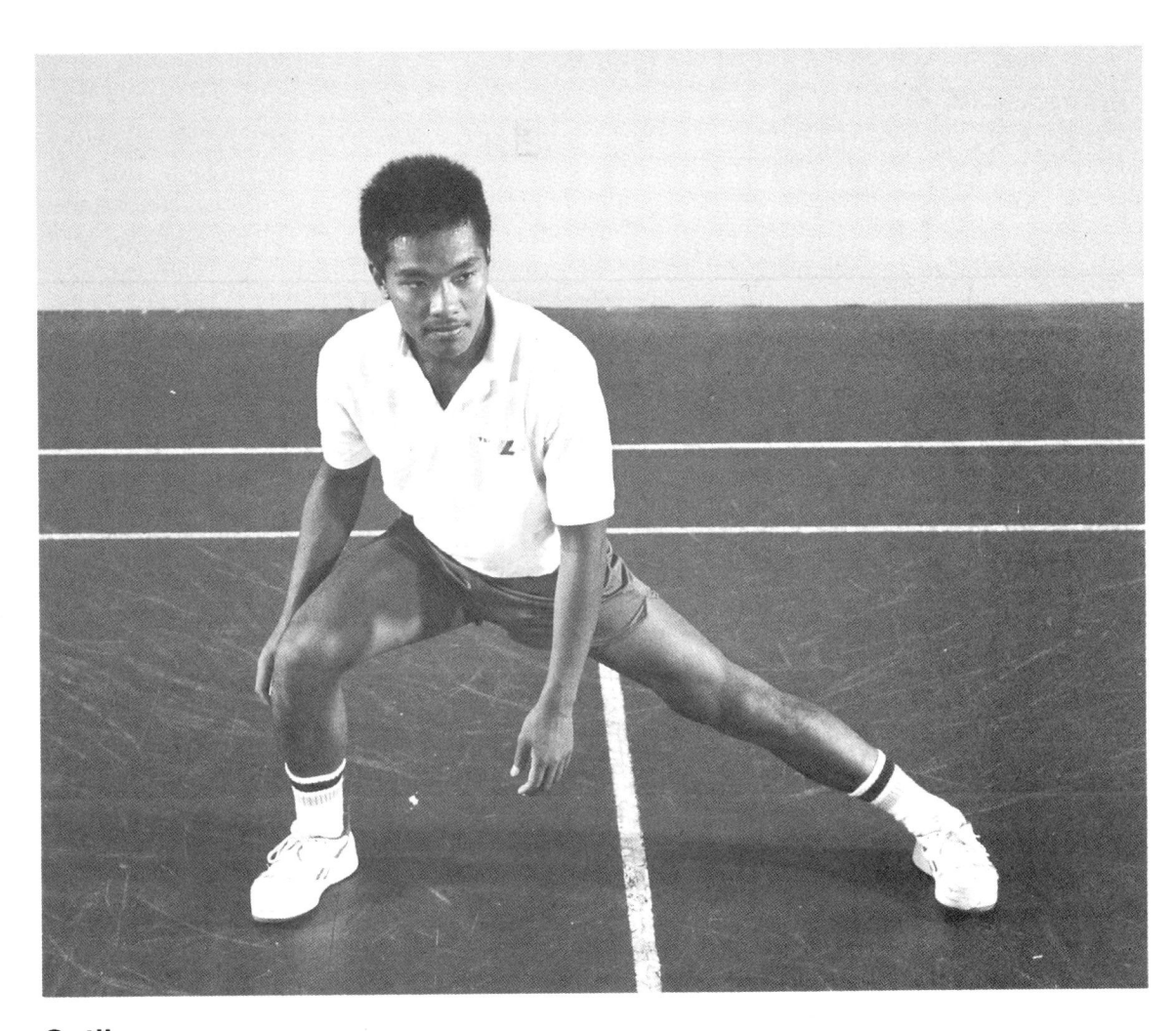

Outline

Setting Goals
Mental Practice
    Imagery or Visualization
    Relaxation
Checklist for Learning to Relax
    Concentration

Physical Conditioning
    Strength
    Flexibility
    Aerobic (Cardiovascular) Conditioning
Summary

Wishing won't make you a better player; only practice will. Some of your practice must take place on the court, learning the physical skills specific to badminton, but you can also work in a gym to condition your body. In addition, you can work at home (and elsewhere) doing mental practice.

Champions in most sports work to condition their minds as well as their bodies in order to realize their full potential. There are so many skills to practice in badminton and there is so much strategy that such mental practice is most appropriate for this sport. Badminton players at any level can use these proven mental and physical skills to increase their abilities.

Setting Goals

Setting goals is essential to improving in any area of life. It is the first step toward success. And the more detailed and precise your goals, the greater your chances are of accomplishing them, since well-defined goals reveal a higher degree of motivation. In addition to vocational goals—such as becoming a doctor—and social goals—such as being a good mate or parent—we can have recreational goals—such as becoming a competent badminton player. If you place sufficient value on this goal, you will take advantage of the on-court and off-court opportunities to improve in the game. You'll practice your fundamentals and strategy on the court. Off the court, you can use mental techniques for visualization, relaxation, and concentration, as well as physical-conditioning exercises to make your body stronger and more flexible.

How quickly do you want to improve? In what areas do you want to improve the most? Quickness, strength or flexibility? Or are you interested in developing additional types of serves? Do you need work on drop shots or smashes? Your greatest needs will determine the goals you set. Make them realistic, and develop a practice schedule for attaining them.

Mental Practice

As mentioned, championship athletes have known for years that mental practice helps their coordination. Only recently, however, have sports psychologists refined the methods of perfecting the mind's contribution to the game.[1]

Imagery or Visualization

Mental imagery or *visualization* are the names given to mental practice. In one type, done from the outside, you picture yourself performing your strokes and serves the correct way—as if you were watching yourself on a videotape. The golfer, Jack Nicklaus calls this "going to the movies." In a second type of mental imagery, done from the inside, you imagine yourself in motion, "feeling" yourself practicing your skills.

When you are mentally experiencing your game, you can practice your strokes, your footwork, your strategy—whatever is giving you trouble. If your service return is a problem, for example, imagine yourself ready for the return.

---

[1] Vealey, Robin S., "Imagery Training for Performance Enhancement," Applied Sports Psychology, edited by Jean Williams (Mountain View, Calif.: Mayfield Publishing, 1986)

Your imaginary opponent hits to your backhand. You feel yourself stepping left and starting your backswing. You watch the shuttle. You step and start your swing, always watching the shuttle. You complete your swing, still watching the shuttle on your racket.

Sadly the average athlete doesn't realize how important mental practice is. The elite of the athletic world, such as those on Olympic teams, does. Russian sports psychologists, who are among the leaders in their field, are advocating that as much as 70 percent of practice time be devoted to mental practice.

Relaxation

Relaxation is another essential of good badminton. Practice breathing deeply before you are ready to serve or receive. If you are tense, your muscles cannot work as quickly and effectively as when you start relaxed.

To learn to get the most out of your deep breathing, try this exercise. Sit quietly in a chair, close your eyes, and concentrate on breathing deeply. You can say to yourself, "Breathe in breathe out," or you can repeat a non-exciting word or syllable, such as "One" or "om." By keeping your mind from active thought as you concentrate on your breathing, you will cause your muscles to relax, and your blood pressure will be reduced. This "not thinking" is the basis for many of the benefits gained from the practice of meditation.

Once you have learned to relax while sitting calmly in a quiet place, you can transfer that ability to the badminton court when tension strikes. You can recognize tension by a tightness around your shoulders, rapid breathing, and possibly a tendency to miss shots that you would normally make. When you notice one of these signs, just close your eyes (during a break in play) and breathe deeply at least three times. If you have learned to relax off the court, you will be able to relax on the court.

Use your relaxation techniques whenever you need them. Some people breathe deeply before each serve. Others use the technique only when they are obviously tense.

Checklist for Learning to Relax

1. Sit in a comfortable chair in a quiet room.
2. Loosen your clothing and close your eyes.
3. Breathe deeply while saying to yourself, "Breathe in, breathe out," or a one-syllable word such as "one." This should help you to block all other thoughts from your mind, including the ones that can cause tension.
4. If other thoughts come into your mind, don't worry. Just get back into your breathing pattern and your repetition of the unexciting phrase or word.

Concentration

Concentration is the third major area of mental concern. In badminton the object of your concentration should be the shuttle. Not watching the shuttle all the way to your racket and while it is on your racket is probably the most common and critical error at every level of badminton. Slow-motion movies show us that most people take their eyes off the shuttle when it is still 4 to 6 feet away from them. They start looking at where they are going to hit it rather than watching the hit. You should continue to watch the spot where you hit the shuttle even after it has left your racket in order to train yourself to keep your eye on the shuttle hitting the racket.

Physical Conditioning

Strength

Strength is essential for most athletic events, including badminton. Leg strength is needed to move quickly to every shot. Abdominal and shoulder strength are essential to hit through the shuttle quickly and effortlessly. And wrist strength is necessary for every shot.

Maximum strength is gained by exhausting your muscles in a few repetitions—one to four. More than that tends to develop muscular endurance rather than strength. Since badminton players need both strength and endurance they should do seven to ten repetitions of an exercise rather than one to four (which would be more beneficial for competitive weight lifters) or more than ten (which would develop only endurance). Three sets of each exercise are recommended, three times per week, with at least a day of rest between each day of work.

Wrist strength—actually, forearm strength—is essential in serving. About half of all beginners lack the necessary strength to swing the racket up and hammer the shuttle down toward the court in a smash. To prepare for the smash, you can do wrist curls with weights or take a dumbbell weighted on

Getting wrist strength by using broom:
For the backhand

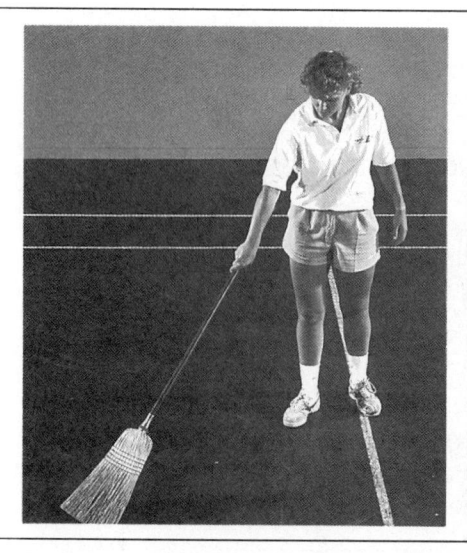

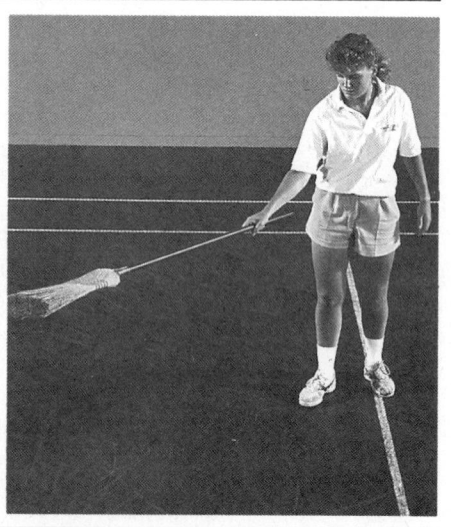

Getting wrist strength by using broom: For the forehand

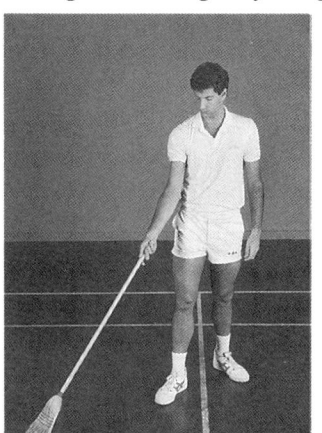

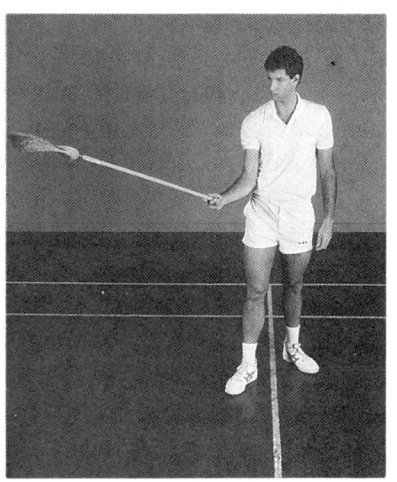

only one end and lift the weighted end. But the simplest way to get sufficient strength quickly is to simply hold the end of a broom, palm up, then raise the broom. You will generally have enough forearm strength to smash after a week of doing this exercise. This can also be done palm down for backhand strength.

Give yourself manual resistance by bending one hand back at the wrist, then pushing against it with the other hand, bring the bent wrist through 180 degrees.

Do the same exercise for the back of your forearm, with your palm down. This will help strengthen your forearm for backhand shots and help prevent *tennis elbow*, the result of playing with weak forearm muscles and tendons.

Using manual resistance to strengthen forearm

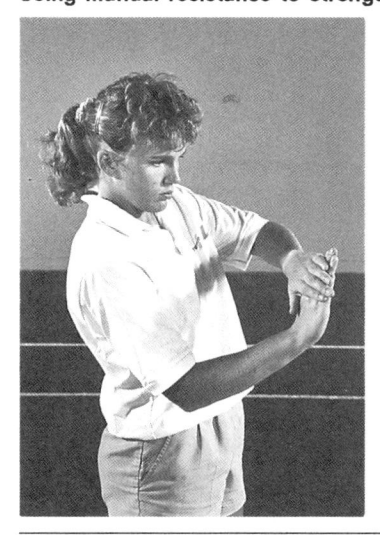

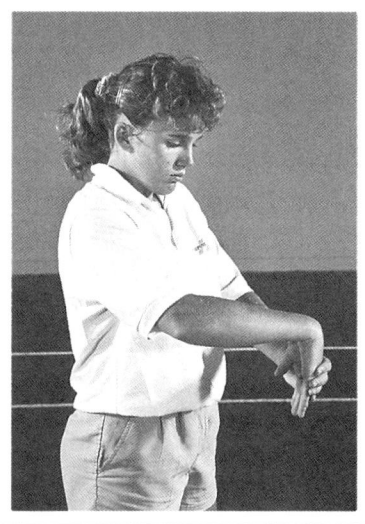

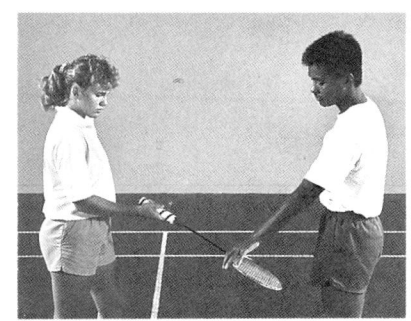

Manual resistance using racket

Standing triceps extension

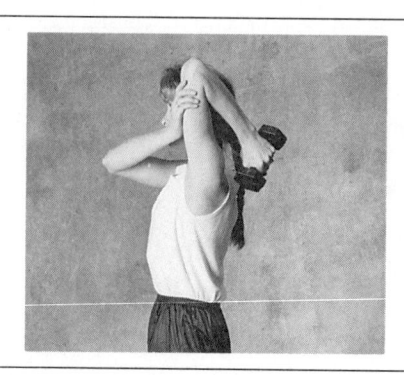

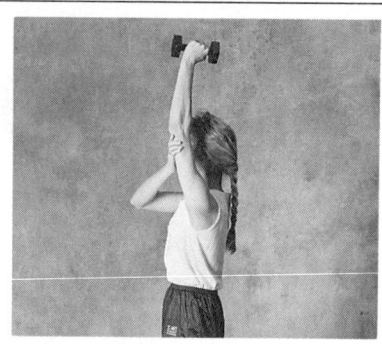

You can give yourself resistance by pushing against the back of your hand and making it work through a full range of motion.

Triceps strength is needed to bring the racket up in the smash. The triceps are reasonably strong in most people, but additional strength can improve your speed in bringing the racket up and hitting through the shuttle. Pushups, bench presses, and French curls are good triceps exercises. Or you can take that same broomstick, hold it at the end, and with your elbow up (as in a smashing action), smash with the broomstick. Not too fast!

Add resistance by bending your right arm, touching your shoulder with your hand. Now use the other hand to push against the wrist of the bent arm as you straighten that arm. This is called *manual resistance* or *dynamic tension*.

Upper back strength is used in hitting the backhand. If you have dumbbells, take one in each hand, bend over, and lift the dumbbells up to your side.

Leg strength can be developed by simply jumping. Or if you have access to weights or a gym, do leg extensions, leg presses, and half-squats.

Lower back strength can be developed with back arches. Lie on the floor face down and arch your back up. Lift your shoulders and knees off the floor.

Triceps strength using broom

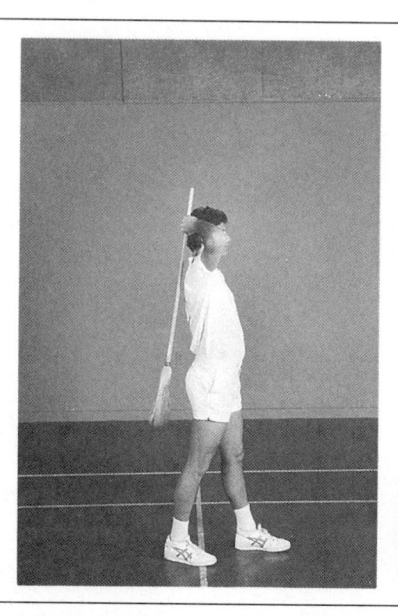

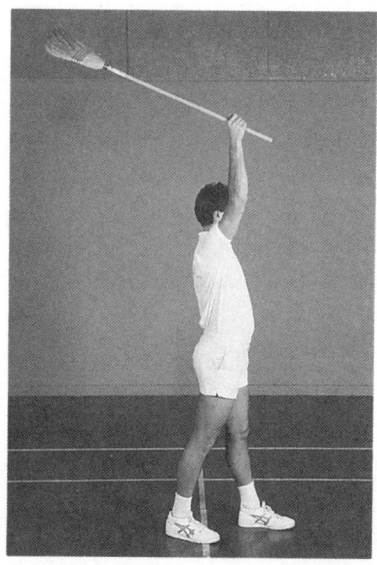

These lower back muscles are often injured in everyday activities, so this exercise should be done throughout your life. This exercise can also be done on a device called a Roman chair.

Abdominal strength is best developed with abdominal curl-ups. With your knees bent and your back on the floor, curl forward, keeping your hips (belt) on the ground. This is another recommended lifelong exercise.

Leg extension on machine

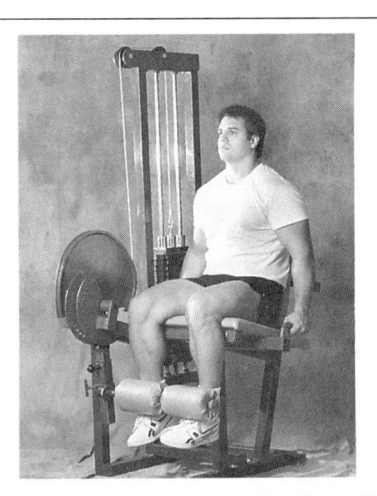

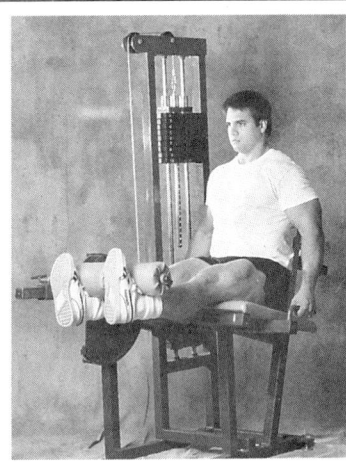

Back arches for lower back strength

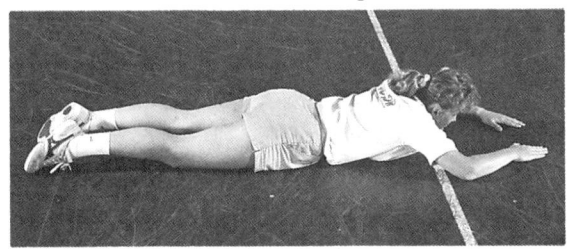

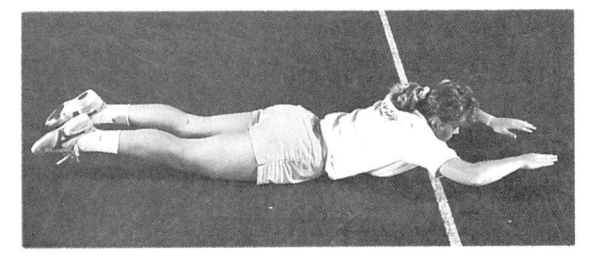

Abdominal curl for abdominal strength

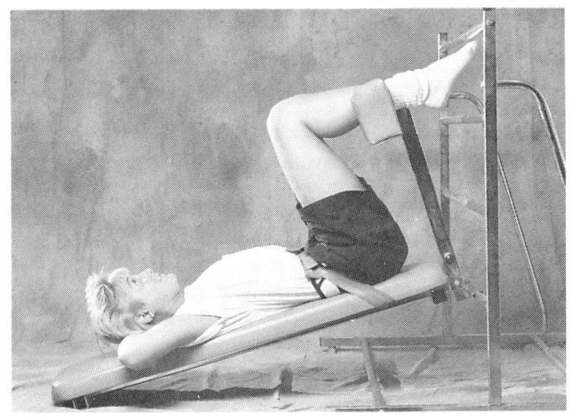

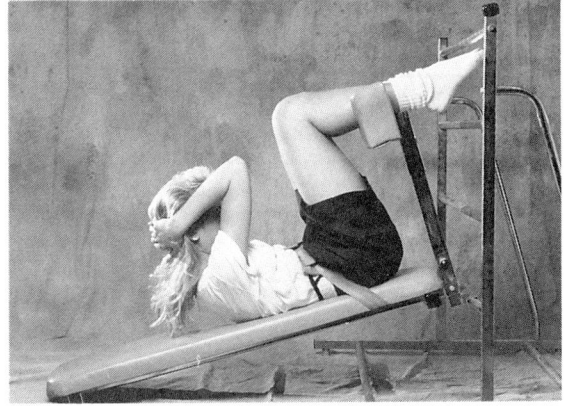

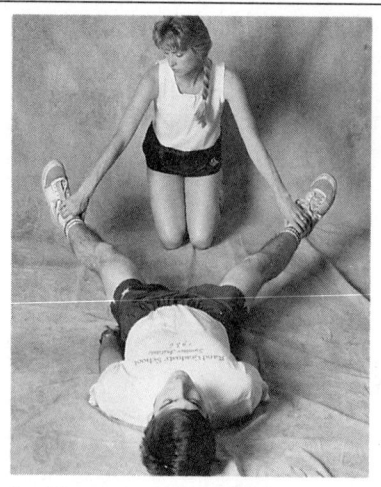

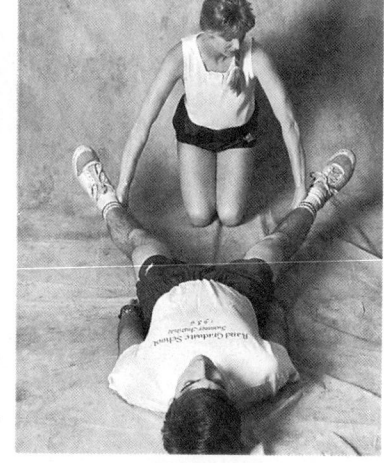

A. Hip abduction with partner **B. Hip adduction with partner**

Groin and side-of-hips strength can be developed on a special machine designed for that purpose or in an exercise that requires a partner. Lie on your back with your legs in the air. Your partner should grasp your ankles. Move your legs out with the partner resisting. Then bring your legs in with your partner again resisting.

Flexibility

You will want good flexibility throughout your body so that you can move smoothly through a full range of motion in every stroke and serve. Do these flexibility exercises before every practice and before every match. They not only make you more flexible, but they warm up the muscles and get them ready to play. In addition, warmed muscles and connective tissue are less likely to sustain injury.

The *upper chest* is stretched by bringing your arms to shoulder level, then pulling them backward as far as they will go. For the *upper back*, bring them as far forward as possible and cross them.

Toe touches for hamstring

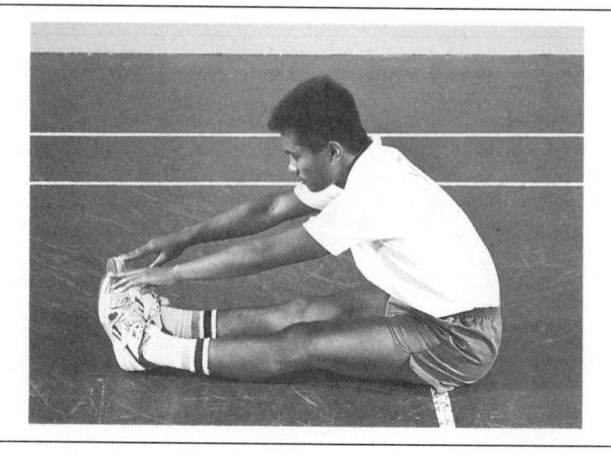

Groin stretch

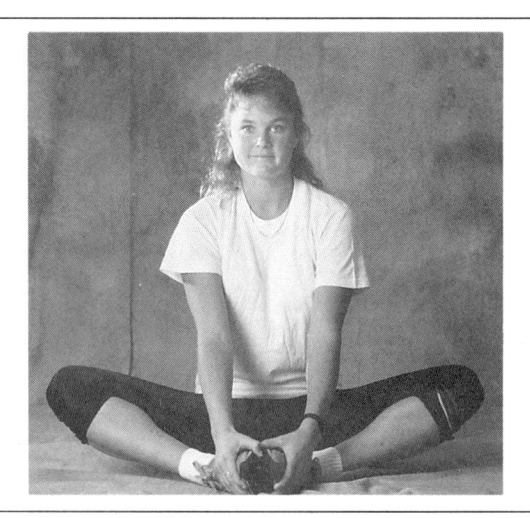

For the *rear of the thighs* (hamstrings), slowly bend down and touch your toes. This exercise is slightly more effective if done in a sitting position.

The *groin area* is stretched by sitting on the floor, putting your feet together and pulling them toward your hips with your hands.

Calf muscles are stretched by standing 3 or 4 feet from a wall or fence and leaning on the support. With your legs straight and your feet flat on the floor,

Thigh and groin stretch

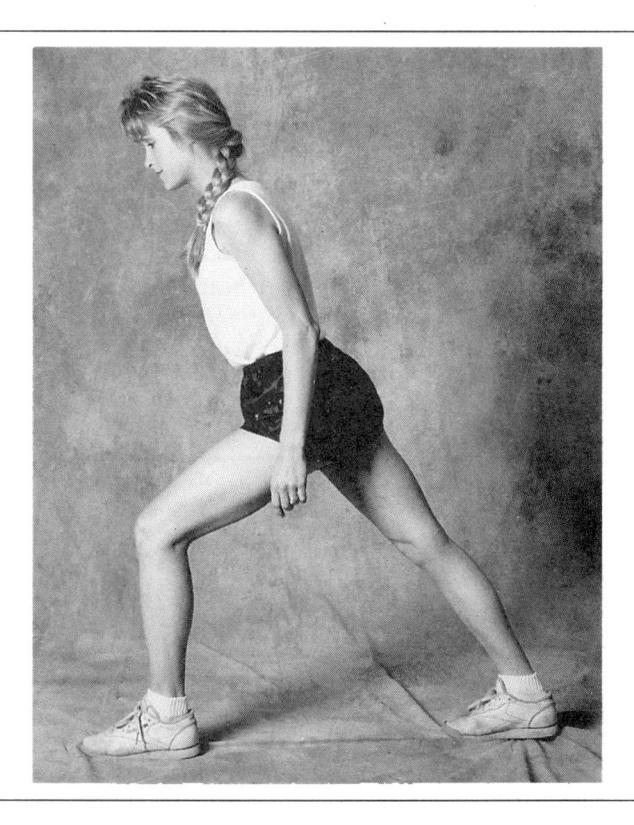

Abdominal twists

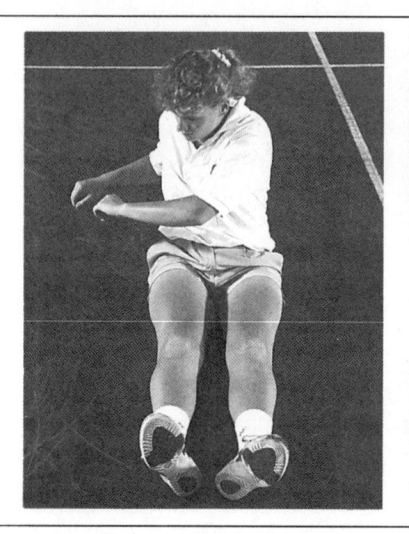

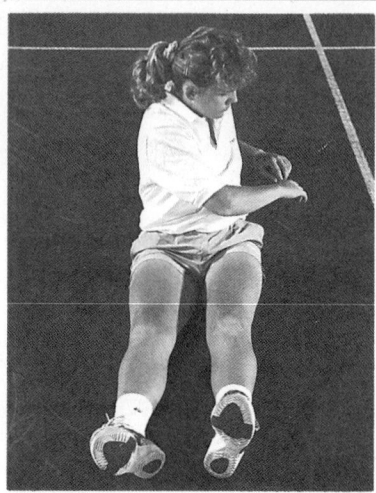

lower your hips until you feel the stretch. Do every stretch slowly and hold for at least 6 to 20 seconds.

Abdominal muscles are stretched by slowly twisting and then bending sideways.

Aerobic (Cardiovascular) Conditioning

To improve your heart's ability to deliver oxygen to your muscles, you need to reach a target-level heart rate and maintain it for 20 to 30 minutes every other day. The target-level range is determined by subtracting your age from the number 220, then taking 65 to 85 percent of the resulting number. So if you are 20 years old, your first calculation would be 220 - 20 = 200. Your second calculation would be 200 x .65 = 130 (the lower range). The third calculation would be 200 x .85 = 170 (the upper range). Your target heart rate is therefore between 130 and 170 heart beats per minute.

There are many ways to exercise aerobically. You can run, skip rope, cycle, or play continuous badminton. In continuous badminton, you keep running. You run while you rally. You run to pick up a shuttle. You run back to the home-base position, then get the shuttle in play.

You can also condition yourself aerobically by playing imaginary badminton against an imaginary partner with an imaginary shuttle. Practice your footwork, your overhand shots, and your underhand shots this way.

Summary

1. A competent badminton player makes use of his or her maximum mental and physical potential. This involves mental and physical practice both on and off the court.
2. Mental conditioning includes
    - Imagery—in which you visualize yourself executing techniques and performing in game situations.

- Relaxation—in which you breathe deeply and disengage your mind from active thinking in order to relieve tension and thus perform at a higher level.
- Concentration—in which you focus on a certain aspect of the game. A beginner may concentrate on perfecting the backswing or follow-through. An intermediate or advanced player will concentrate on keeping his or her eyes on the bird.

3. Goal setting is important for all areas of our lives, including improvement in badminton.
4. To fulfill your potential as a badminton player, you must develop adequate strength, flexibility, and cardiovascular endurance.
5. For badminton, strength and flexibility are most important in the following areas: thighs, groin, upper chest, back, wrists, triceps, legs, and abdominals.
6. Proper stretching exercises not only prepare the muscles to react to their maximum potential but also reduce the chances of muscular and connective-tissue injuries.

APPENDIX A

Laws of Badminton*

Laws

1. **COURT**
    1.1 The court shall be a rectangle and laid out as in the following Diagram "A" (except in the case provided for in law 1.5) and to the measurements there shown, defined by lines 40 mm wide.
    1.2 The lines shall be easily distinguishable and preferably be colored white or yellow.
    1.3.1 To show the zone in which a shuttle of correct pace lands when tested (Law 4.4), an additional four marks 40 mm by 40 mm may be made inside each side line for singles of the right service court, 530 mm and 990 mm from the back boundary line.
    1.3.2 In making these marks, their width shall be within the measurement given, *i.e.*, the marks will be from 530 mm to 570 mm and from 950 mm to 990 mm from the outside of the back boundary line.
    1.4 All lines form part of the area which they define.
    1.5 Where space does not permit the marking out of a court for doubles, a court may be marked out for singles only as shown in Diagram "B." The back boundary lines become also the long service lines, and the posts or the strips of material representing them (Law 2.2), shall be placed on the side lines.

2. **POSTS**
    2.1 The posts shall be 1.55 meters in height from the surface of the court. They shall be sufficiently firm to remain vertical and keep the net strained as provided in Law 3, and shall be placed on the doubles side lines as shown in Diagram "A."
    2.2 Where it is not practicable to have posts on the side lines, some method must be used to indicate the position of the side lines where they pass under the net, e.g., by the use of thin posts or strips of material 40 mm wide, fixed to the side lines and rising vertically to the net cord.
    2.3 On a court marked for doubles, the posts or strips of material representing the posts shall be placed on the side lines for doubles, irrespective of whether singles or doubles is being played.

3. **NET**
    3.1 The net shall be made of fine cord of dark color and even thickness with a mesh not less than 15 mm and not more than 20 mm.

---

*Excerpted and reprinted from *Official Rules of Play*, © 1987, pps. 21–49, with permission from the United States Badminton Association.

Diagram A

Court dimensions:
- 40 mm / 420 mm / 40 mm
- 2,530 m | 40 mm | 2,530 m | 40 mm / 420 mm / 40 mm
- Back boundary (base) line
- 40 mm
- 720 mm — Also long service line for singles / Long service line for doubles
- 40 mm
- Doubles side line
- 3,880 m — Right service court | Center line | Left service court
- 40 mm
- 1,980 m — Short service line
- Net — 13,400 m
- Post .... Post
- 1,980 m
- 40 mm — Short service line
- Singles side line
- 3,880 m — Left service court | Center line | Right service court | Singles side line
- 40 mm
- 720 mm — Long service line for doubles
- 40 mm — Back boundary (base) line / Also long service line for singles
- 6.100 m

Note: Court can be used for both singles and doubles play.

Diagonal length of full court = 14.723 m

Optional testing marks for doubles court (see Law 1.3)

Right service court

N.B. measurement of marks 40 mm by 40 mm

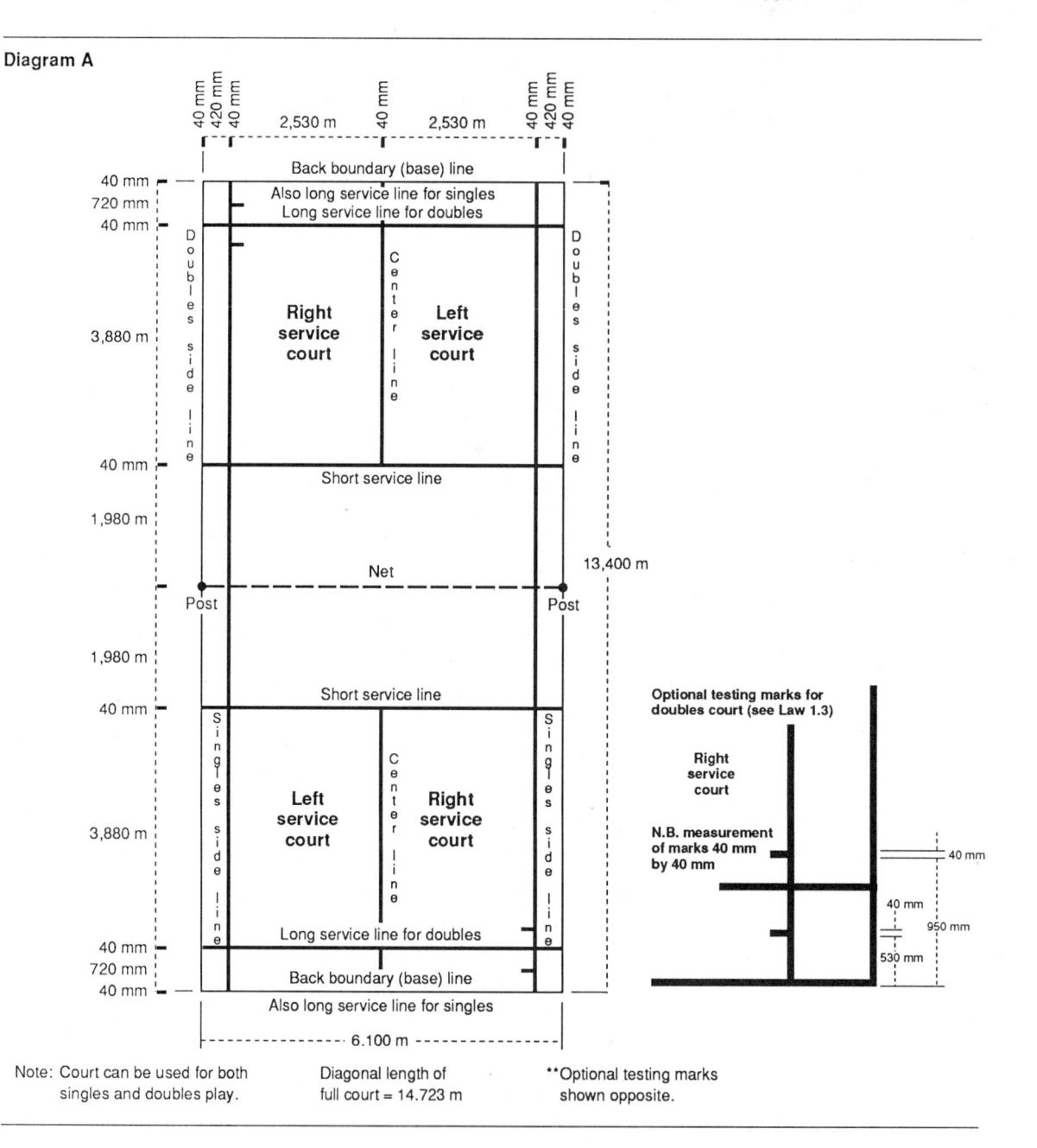

- 40 mm
- 40 mm
- 950 mm
- 530 mm

**Optional testing marks shown opposite.

3.2 The net shall be 760 mm in depth.

3.3 The top of the net shall be edged with a 75 mm white tape doubled over a cord or cable running through the tape. This tape must rest upon the cord or cable.

3.4 The cord or cable shall be of sufficient size and weight to be firmly stretched flush with the top of the posts.

APPENDIX A 115

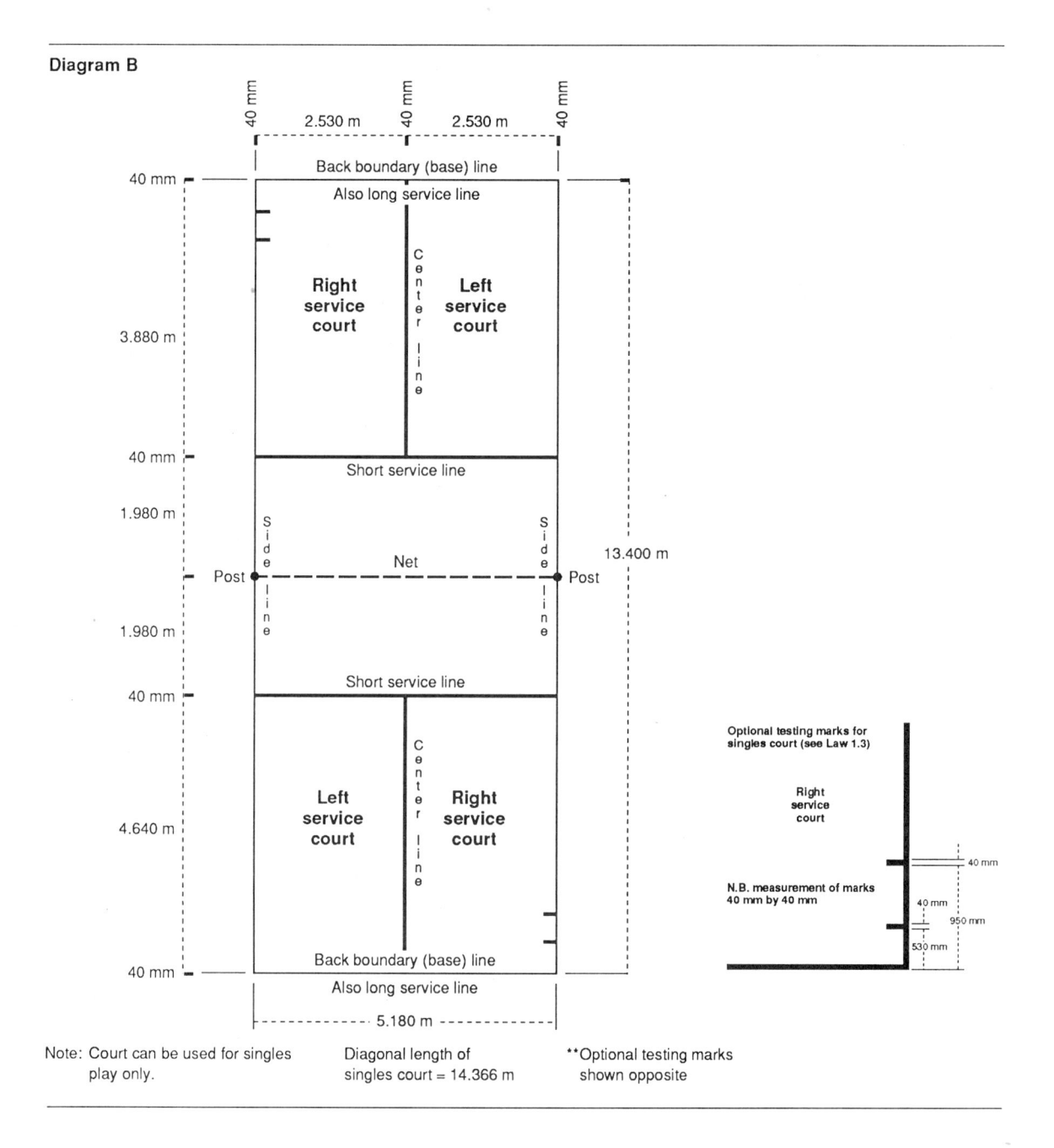

Diagram B

[Badminton court diagram with the following labeled measurements and features:]

- 40 mm, 2.530 m, 40 mm, 2.530 m, 40 mm (across the top)
- Back boundary (base) line / Also long service line
- 40 mm
- Right service court | Center line | Left service court
- 3.880 m
- 40 mm
- Short service line
- 1.980 m
- Side line — Net — Side line
- Post — — — Post
- 13.400 m
- 1.980 m
- Short service line
- 40 mm
- Left service court | Center line | Right service court
- 4.640 m
- 40 mm
- Back boundary (base) line / Also long service line
- 5.180 m

Note: Court can be used for singles play only.

Diagonal length of singles court = 14.366 m

**Optional testing marks shown opposite

Optional testing marks for singles court (see Law 1.3)

Right service court

N.B. measurement of marks 40 mm by 40 mm

40 mm
40 mm
950 mm
530 mm

3.5 The top of the net from the surface of the court shall be 1.524 meters at the center of the court and 1.55 meters over the side lines for doubles.

3.6 There shall be no gaps between the ends of the net and the posts. If necessary, the full depth of the net should be tied at the ends.

4. SHUTTLE

Principles

The shuttle may be made from natural and/or synthetic materials. Whatever material the shuttle is made from, the flight characteristics, generally, should be similar to those produced by a natural feathered shuttle with a cork base covered by a thin layer of feather.

Having regard to the Principles:

4.1 *General Design*

    4.1.1 The shuttle shall have 16 feathers fixed in the base.

    4.1.2 The feathers can have a variable length from 64 mm to 70 mm, but in each shuttle they shall be the same length when measured from the tip to the top of the base.

    4.1.3 The tips of the feathers shall form a circle with a diameter from 58 mm to 68 mm.

    4.1.4 The feathers shall be fastened firmly with thread or other suitable material.

    4.1.5 The base shall be:
- 25 mm to 28 mm in diameter
- rounded on the bottom

4.2 *Weight*

The shuttle shall weigh from 4.74 to 5.50 grams.

4.3 *Non-Feathered Shuttle*

    4.3.1 The skirt, or simulation of feathers in synthetic materials, replaces natural feathers.

    4.3.2 The base is described in Law 4.1 5.

    4.3.3 Measurements and weight shall be as in Laws 4.1.2, 4.1.3 and 4.2. However, because of the difference of the specific gravity and behavior of synthetic materials in comparison with feathers, a variation of up to ten percent is acceptable.

4.4 *Shuttle Testing*

    4.4.1 To test a shuttle, use a full underhand stroke which makes contact with the shuttle over the back boundary line. The shuttle shall be hit at an upward angle and in a direction parallel to the side lines.

    4.4.2 A shuttle of correct pace will land not less than 530 mm and not more than 990 mm short of the other back boundary line.

4.5 *Modifications*

Subject to there being no variation in the general design, pace and flight of the shuttle, modifications in the above specifications may be made with the approval of the National Organization concerned:

    4.5.1 in places where atmospheric conditions due to either altitude or climate make the standard shuttle unsuitable; or

APPENDIX A

    4.5.2   if special circumstances exist which make it otherwise necessary in the interests of the game.

5. RACKET

5.1   The hitting surface of the racket shall be flat and consist of a pattern of crossed strings connected to a frame and either alternately interlaced or bonded where they cross. The stringing pattern shall be generally uniform and, in particular, not less dense in the center than in any other area.

5.2   The frame of the racket, including the handle, shall not exceed 680 mm in overall length and 230 mm in overall width.

5.3   The overall length of the head shall not exceed 290 mm.

5.4   The strung surface shall not exceed 280 mm in overall length and 220 mm in overall width.

5.5   The racket:

    5.5.1   shall be free of attached objects and protrusions, other than those utilized solely and specifically to limit or prevent wear and tear, or vibration, or to distribute weight, or to secure the handle by cord to the player's hand, and which are reasonable in size and placement for such purposes; and

    5.52   shall be free of any device which makes it possible for a player to change materially the shape of the racket.

6. APPROVED EQUIPMENT

The International Badminton Federation shall rule on any question of whether any racket, shuttle or equipment or any prototypes used in the playing of Badminton complies with the specifications or is otherwise approved or not approved for play. Such ruling may be undertaken on the Federation's initiative or upon application by any party with a bona fide interest therein including any player, equipment manufacturer or National Organization or member thereof.

7. PLAYERS

7.1   "Player" applies to all those taking part in a match.

7.2   The game shall be played, in the case of doubles, by two players a side, or in the case of singles, by one player a side.

7.3   The side having the right to serve shall be called the serving side, and the opposing side shall be called the receiving side.

8. TOSS

8.1   Before commencing play, the opposing sides shall toss and the side winning the toss shall exercise the choice in either Law 8.1.1 or Law 8.1.2.

    8.1.1   To serve or receive first.

    8.1.2   To start play at one end of the court or the other.

8.2   The side losing the toss shall then exercise the remaining choice.

9. SCORING

9.1 The opposing sides shall play the best of three games unless otherwise arranged.

9.2 Only the serving side can add a point to its score.

9.3 In doubles and Men's singles a game is won by the first side to score 15 points, except as provided in Law 9.6.

9.4 In Ladies' singles a game is won by the first side to score 11 points, except as provided in Law 9.6.

9.5.1 If the score becomes 13 all or 14 all (9 all or 10 all in Ladies' singles), the side which first scored 13 or 14 (9 or 10) shall have the choice of "setting" or "not setting" the game (Law 9.6).

9.5.2 This choice can only be made when the score is first reached and must be made before the next service is delivered.

9.5.3 The relevant side (Law 9.5.1) is given the opportunity to set at 14 all (10 all in Ladies' singles) despite any previous decision not to set by that side or the opposing side at 13 all (9 all in Ladies' singles).

9.6 If the game has been set, the score is called "Love All" and the side first scoring the set number of points (Law 9.6.12 to 9.6.4) wins the game.

  9.6.1 13 all setting to 5 points
  9.6.2 14 all setting to 3 points
  9.6.3 9 all setting to 3 points
  9.6.4 10 all setting to 2 points

9.7 The side winning a game serves first in the next game.

10. CHANGE OF ENDS

10.1 Players shall change ends:

  10.1.1 at the end of the first game;
  10.1.2 prior to the beginning of the third game (if any); and
  10.1.3 in the third game, or in a one game match, when the leading score reaches:
  - 6 in a game of 11 points
  - 8 in a game of 15 points

10.2 When players omit to change ends as indicated by Law 10.1, they shall do so immediately the mistake is discovered and the existing score shall stand.

11 SERVICE

11.1 In a correct service:

  11.1.1 neither side shall cause undue delay to the delivery of the service;
  11.1.2 the server and receiver shall stand within diagonally opposite service courts without touching the boundary lines of these service courts; some part of both feet of the server and receiver must remain in contact with the surface of the court in a stationary position until the service is delivered (Law 11.4);

APPENDIX A

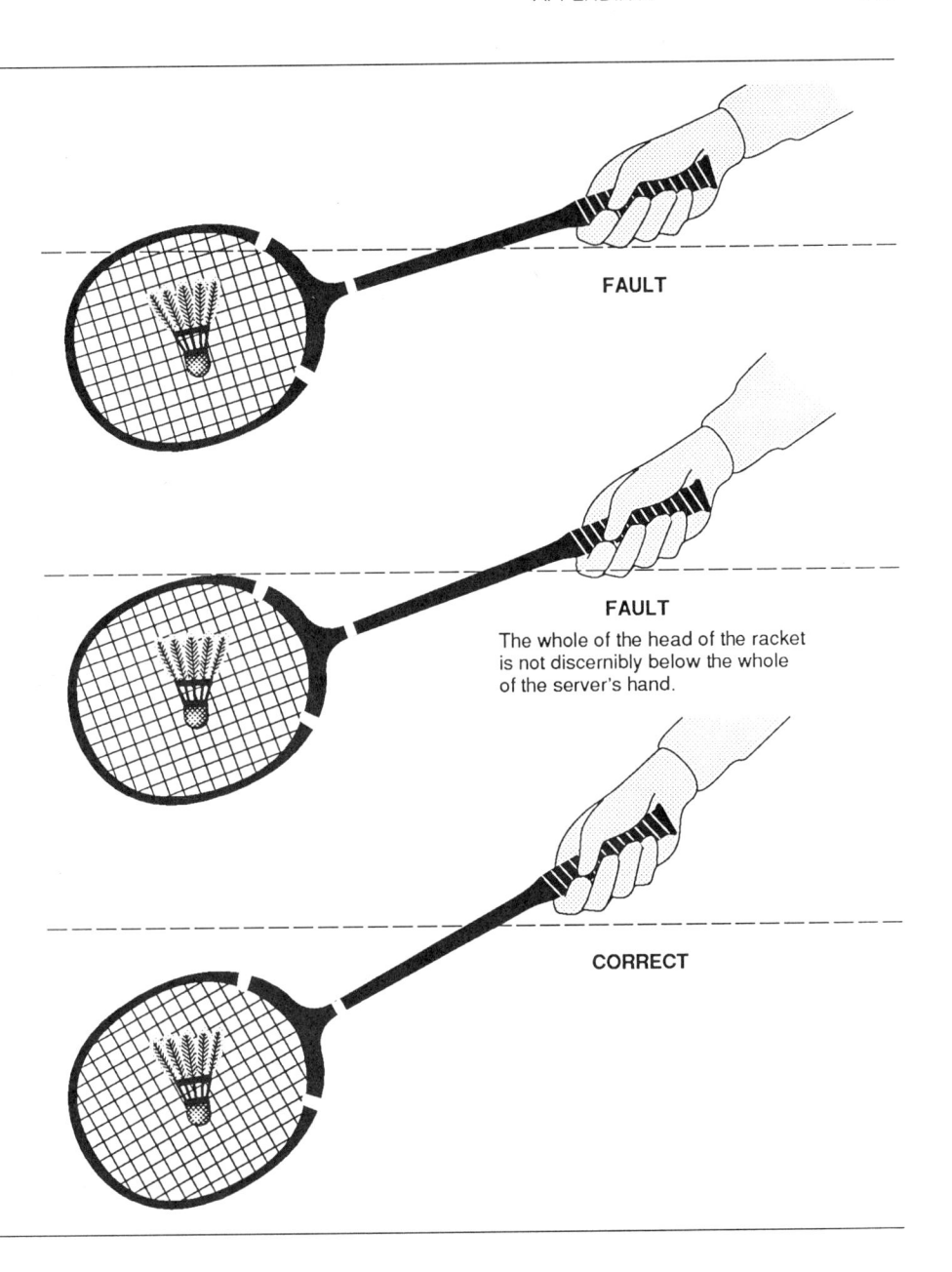

FAULT

FAULT

The whole of the head of the racket is not discernibly below the whole of the server's hand.

CORRECT

11.1.3 the server's racket shall initially hit the base of the shuttle while the whole of the shuttle is below the server's waist;

11.1.4 the shaft of the server's racket at the instant of hitting the shuttle shall be pointing in a downward direction to such an extent that the whole of the head of the racket is discernibly below the whole of the server's hand holding the racket;

11.1.5 the movement of the server's racket must continue forwards after the start of the service (Law 11.2) until the service is delivered; and

11.1.6   the flight of the shuttle shall be upwards from the server's racket to pass over the net, so that, if not intercepted, it falls in the receiver's service court.

11.2   Once the players have taken their positions, the first forward movement of the server's racket is the start of the service.

11.3   The server shall not serve before the receiver is ready, but the receiver shall be considered to have been ready if a return of service is attempted.

11.4   The service is delivered when, once started (Law 11.2), the shuttle is hit by the server's racket or the shuttle lands on the floor.

11.5   In doubles, the partners, may take up any positions which do not unsight the opposing server or receiver.

12. SINGLES

12.1   The players shall serve from, and receive in, their respective right service courts when the server has not scored or has scored an even number of points in that game.

12.2   The players shall serve from, and receive in, their respective left service courts when the server has scored an odd number of points in that game.

12.3   If a game is set, the total points scored by the server in that game shall be used to apply Laws 12.1 and 12.2.

12.4   The shuttle is hit alternately by the server and the receiver until a "fault" is made or the shuttle ceases to be in play.

12.5.1   If the receiver makes a "fault" or the shuttle ceases to be in play because it touches the surface of the court inside the receiver's court, the server scores a point. The server then serves again from the alternate service court.

12.5.2   If the server makes a "fault" or the shuttle ceases to be in play because it touches the surface of the court inside the server's court, the server loses the right to continue serving, and the receiver then becomes the server, with no point scored by either player.

13. DOUBLES

13.1   At the start of a game, and each time a side gains the right to serve, the service shall be delivered from the right service court.

13.2   Only the receiver shall return the service: should the shuttle touch or be hit by the receiver's partner, the serving side scores a point.

13.3.1   After the service is returned, the shuttle is hit by either player of the serving side and then by either player of the receiving side, and so on, until the shuttle ceases to be in play.

13.3.2   After the service is returned, a player may hit the shuttle from any position on that player's side of the net.

13.4.1   If the receiving side makes a "fault" or the shuttle ceases to be in play because it touches the surface of the court inside the receiving side's court, the serving side scores a point, and the server serves again.

13.4.2 If the serving side makes a "fault" or the shuttle ceases to be in play because it touches the surface of the court inside the serving side's court, the server loses the right to continue serving, with no point scored by either side.

13.5.1 The player who serves at the start of any game shall serve from, or receive in, the right service court when that player's side has not scored or has scored an even number of points in that game, and the left service court otherwise.

13.5.2 The player who receives at the start of any game shall receive in, or serve from, the right service court when that player's side has not scored or has scored an even number of points in that game, and the left service court otherwise.

13.5.3 The reverse pattern applies to the partners.

13.5.4 If a game is set, the total points scored by a side in that game shall be used to apply Laws 13.5.1 to 13.5.3.

13.6 Service in any turn of serving shall be delivered from alternate service courts, except as provided in Laws 14 and 16.

13.7 The right to serve passes consecutively from the initial server in any game to the initial receiver in that game, and then consecutively from that player to that player's partner and then to one of the opponents and then the opponent's partner, and so on.

13.8 No player shall serve out of turn, receive out of turn, or receive two consecutive services in the same game, except as provided in Laws 14 and 16.

13.9 Either player of the winning side may serve first in the next game and either player of the losing side may receive.

14. SERVICE COURT ERRORS

14.1 A service court error has been made when a player:
- 14.1.1 has served out of turn;
- 14.1.2 has served from the wrong service court; or
- 14.1.3 standing in the wrong service court, was prepared to receive the service and it has been delivered.

14.2 When a service court error has been made, then:
- 14.2.1 if the error is discovered before the next service is delivered, it is a "let" unless only one side was at fault and lost the rally, in which case the error shall not be corrected.
- 14.2.2 if the error is not discovered before the next service is delivered, the error shall not be corrected.

14.3 If there is a "let" because of a service court error, the rally is replayed with the error corrected.

14.4 If a service court error is not to be corrected, play in that game shall proceed without changing the players' new service courts (nor, when relevant, the new order of serving).

15. FAULTS

It is a "fault":

- 15.1 if a service is not correct (Law 11.1);
- 15.2 if the server, in attempting to serve, misses the shuttle;
- 15.3 if after passing over the net on service, the shuttle is caught in or on the net;
- 15.4 if in play, the shuttle;
  - 15.4.1 lands outside the boundaries of the court;
  - 15.4.2 passes through or under the net;
  - 15.4.3 fails to pass the net;
  - 15.4.4 touches the roof, ceiling, or side walls;
  - 15.4.5 touches the person or dress of a player; or
  - 15.4.6 touches any other object or person outside the immediate surroundings of the court;

    (Where necessary on account of the structure of the building, the local badminton authority may, subject to the right of veto of its National Organization, make bye-laws dealing with cases in which a shuttle touches an obstruction).

- 15.5 if, when in play, the initial point of contact with the shuttle is not on the striker's side of the net. (The striker may, however, follow the shuttle over the net with the racket in the course of a stroke).
- 15.6 if, when the shuttle is in play, a player:
  - 15.6.1 touches the net or its supports with racket, person or dress;
  - 15.6.2 invades an opponent's court with racket or person in any degree except as permitted in Law 15.5; or
  - 15.6.3 prevents an opponent from making a legal stroke where the shuttle is followed over the net;
- 15.7 if, in play, a player deliberately distracts an opponent by any action such as shouting or making gestures;
- 15.8 if, in play, the shuttle;
  - 15.8.1 be caught and held on the racket and then slung during the execution of a stroke;
  - 15.8.2 be hit twice in succession by the same player with two strokes; or
  - 15.8.3 be hit by a player and the player's partner successively; or
- 15.9 if a player is guilty of flagrant, repeated or persistent offenses under Law 18.

16. LETS

"Let" is called by the Umpire, or by a player (if there is not Umpire) to halt play.

- 16.1 A "let" may be given for any unforeseen or accidental occurrence.
- 16.2 If a shuttle, after passing over the net, is caught in or on the net, it is a "let" except during service.

16.3 If during service, the receiver and server are both faulted at the same time, it shall be a "let."

16.4 If the server serves before the receiver is ready it shall be a "let."

16.5 If during play, the shuttle disintegrates and the base completely separates from the rest of the shuttle, it shall be a "let."

16.6 If a Line Judge is unsighted and the Umpire is unable to make a decision, it shall be a "let."

16.7 When a "let" occurs, the play since the last service shall not count, and the player who served shall serve again, except when Law 14 is applicable.

17. SHUTTLE NOT IN PLAY

A shuttle is not in play when:

17.1 it strikes the net and remains attached there or suspended on top;

17.2 it strikes the net or post and starts to fall towards the surface of the court on the striker's side of the net;

17.3 it hits the surface of the court; or

17.4 a "fault" or "let" has occurred.

18. CONTINUOUS PLAY, MISCONDUCT, PENALTIES

18.1 Play shall be continuous from the first service until the match is concluded, except as allowed in Laws 18.2 and 18.3.

18.2 An interval not exceeding 5 minutes is allowed between the second and third games of all matches in all of the following situations:

    18.2.1 in international competitive events;
    18.2.2 in IBF sanctioned events; and
    18.2.3 in all other matches (unless the National Organization has previously published a decision not to allow such an interval).

18.3 When necessitated by circumstances not within the control of the players, the Umpire may suspend play for such a period as the Umpire may consider necessary. If play be suspended, the existing score shall stand and play be resumed from that point.

18.4 Under no circumstances shall play be suspended to enable a player to recover his strength or wind, or to receive instruction or advice.

18.5.1 Except in the intervals provided in Laws 18.2 and 18.3, no player shall be permitted to receive advice during a match.

18.5.2 Except at the conclusion of a match, no player shall leave the court without the Umpire's consent.

18.6 The Umpire shall be the sole judge of any suspension of play.

18.7 A player shall not:

    18.7.1 deliberately cause suspension of play;
    18.7.2 deliberately interfere with the speed of the shuttle;

	18.7.3	behave in an offensive manner; or
	18.7.4	be guilty of misconduct not otherwise covered by the Laws of Badminton.

18.8 The Umpire shall administer any breach of Law 18.4, 18.5 or 18.7 by:

    18.8.1   issuing a warning to the offending side;
    18.8.2   faulting the offending side, if previously warned; or
    18.8.3   in cases of flagrant offense or persistent offenses, faulting the offending side and reporting the offending side immediately to the Referee, who shall have the power to disqualify.

18.9 Where a Referee has not been appointed, the responsible official shall have the power to disqualify.

19. OFFICIALS AND APPEALS

19.1 The Referee is in overall charge of the tournament or event of which a match forms part.

19.2 The Umpire, where appointed, is in charge of the match, the court and its immediate surrounds. The Umpire shall report to the Referee. In the absence of a Referee, the Umpire shall report instead to the responsible official.

19.3 The Service Judge shall call service faults made by the server should they occur (Law 11).

19.4 A Line Judge shall indicate whether a shuttle is "in" or "out."

An Umpire shall:

19.5 uphold and enforce the Laws of Badminton and, especially call a "fault" or "let" should either occur, without appeal being made by the players;

19.6 give a decision on any appeal regarding a point of dispute, if made before the next service is delivered;

19.7 ensure players and spectators are kept informed of the progress of the match;

19.8 appoint or remove Line Judges or a Service Judge in consultation with the Referee;

19.9 not overrule the decisions of Line Judges and the Service Judge on points of fact;

19.10.1 where another court official is not appointed, arrange for their duties to be carried out;

19.10.2 where an appointed official is unsighted, carry out the official's duties or play a "let";

19.11 decide upon any suspension of play;

19.12 record and report to the Referee all matters in relation to Law 18; and

19.13 Take to the Referee all unsatisfied appeals on questions of Law only.

(Such appeals must be made before the next service is delivered, or, if at the end of a game, before the side that appeals has left the court.)

Appendices to the Laws of Badminton

APPENDIX 1

Imperial measurements

The Laws express all measurements in meters or millimeters. Imperial measurements are acceptable and for the purposes of the Laws the following table of equivalence should be used:

15 millimeters	⅛ inch
20 millimeters	¼ inch
25 millimeters	1 inch
28 millimeters	1 ⅛ inches
40 millimeters	1 ½ inches
58 millimeters	2 ¼ inches
64 millimeters	2 ½ inches
68 millimeters	2 ⅝ inches
70 millimeters	2 ¼ inches
75 millimeters	3 inches
220 millimeters	8 ⅝ inches
230 millimeters	9 inches
280 millimeters	11 inches
290 millimeters	11 ⅜ inches
380 millimeters	1 foot 3 inches
420 millimeters	1 foot 4 ½ inches
490 millimeters	1 foot 7 ½ inches
530 millimeters	1 foot 9 inches
570 millimeters	1 foot 10 ½ inches
680 millimeters	2 feet 2 ¼ inches
720 millimeters	2 feet 4 ½ inches
760 millimeters	2 feet 6 inches
950 millimeters	3 feet 1 ½ inches
990 millimeters	3 feet 3 inches
1.524 meters	5 feet
1.55 meters	5 feet 1 inch
2.53 meters	8 feet 3 ¼ inches
3.88 meters	12 feet 9 inches
4.64 meters	15 feet 3 inches
5.18 meters	17 feet
6.1 meters	20 feet
13.4 meters	44 feet

APPENDIX 2

Handicap matches

In handicap matches, the following variations in the Laws apply:

1. "Setting" is not permitted (i.e., Laws 9.5 and 9.6 do not apply).
2. Law 10.1.3 will be amended to read:
    "In the third game, and in a one game match, when one side has scored half the total number of points required to win the game (the next higher number being taken in case of fractions)."

APPENDIX 3

Games of other than 11 or 15 points

It is permissible to play one game of 21 points by prior arrangement. In this case the following variations in Laws 9.3, 9.5.1, 9.5.3 and 9.6 apply:

Replace "13," "14" and "15 by "19," "20" and "21" respectively.
To Law 10.1.3 shall be added "• 11 in a game of 21 points."

APPENDIX 4

Vocabulary

This Appendix lists the standard vocabulary that should be used by Umpires to control a match.

1. *Announcements and Introductions*
    - 1.1   "Ladies and Gentlemen," this is:
        - 1.1.1   the semi-final, or final, of Men's Singles, etc. or
        - 1.1.2   the first singles of the Thomas Cup (Uber Cup) tie between _____(Country) and _____(Country)
    - 1.2   On my right _____(Name and Country)
      On my left _____(Name and Country)
    - 1.3   _____ to serve _____ to receive.

2. *Start of Match and Calling the Score*
    - 2.1   "Love all; play"
    - 2.2   "Service Over"
    - 2.3   "Second Server"
    - 2.4   "_____ Game Point _____" e.g. "14 game point 6"
    - 2.5   "_____ Match Point _____" e.g. "14 match point 8"
    - 2.6   "_____ Game Point _____" e.g. "2 game point all"
    - 2.7   "Game won by _____(and the score)_____"
    - 2.8   "Second game won by _____(and the score)_____"
    - 2.9   "Are you setting?"
        - 2.9.1   "Setting 2 points; Love-all"
        - 2.9.2   "Setting 3 points; Love-all"
        - 2.9.3   "Setting 5 points; Love-all"
    - 2.10   "Game not set" (Call score "9-all, play"; "13-all, play", etc.)
    - 2.11   "One game all"
    - 2.12   "Court ____ a five minute interval has been claimed"
    - 2.13.1   "Court ____ two minutes remaining."
    - 2.13.2   "Court ____ one minute remaining."

3. *General Communication*
    - 3.1   "Are you ready?"
    - 3.2   "Come here please"

	3.3	"Is the shuttle O.K.?
	3.4	"Test the shuttle" (only for wobble, NOT speed)
	3.5	"Change the shuttle"
	3.6	"Do NOT change the shuttle"
	3.7	"Play a "let"
	3.8	"Change ends, please"
	3.9	"You served out of turn"
	3.10	"You received out of turn"
	3.11	"You must not interfere with the speed of the shuttle"
	3.12	"The shuttle touched you"
	3.13	"You touched the net"
	3.14	"You are standing in the wrong court"
	3.15	"You invaded your opponent's court"
	3.16	"You obstructed your opponent"
	3.17	"Fault—receiver"
	3.18	"Service fault called"
	3.19	"Play must be continuous"
	3.20	"Play is suspended"
	3.21	_____(name of player) "Warning for misconduct"
	3.22	_____(name of player) "Fault for misconduct"
	3.23	"Fault"
	3.24	"Out"
	3.25	"Line Judge—signal please"
	3.26	"Service Judge—signal please"
	3.27	"First server"
	3.28	"Wipe the court"
4.	End of Match	
	4.1	"Match won by _____" (In team event, use name of country)

5. Scoring

0—Love	10—Ten
1—One	11—Eleven
2—Two	12—Twelve
3—Three	13—Thirteen
4—Four	14—Fourteen
5—Five	15—Fifteen
6—Six	16—Sixteen
7—Seven	17—Seventeen
8—Eight	18—Eighteen
9—Nine	

APPENDIX 5

Badminton for disabled people

The following amended Laws of Badminton are applicable to the various categories of disabled people as listed:

a. AMBULANT (No change in the Laws)
   Persons requiring no mechanical aid to perambulation.

b. SEMI-AMBULANT
   Persons capable of erect perambulation but only with mechanical aid such as:

   crutch(es)
   stick(s)
   support frame
   leg braces(s)
   artificial leg(s)

c. NON-AMBULANT
   Persons whose disabilities dictate that they adopt a sedentary posture using such support as:

   chair
   wheel-chair
   stool

The table below shows the changes to Laws.

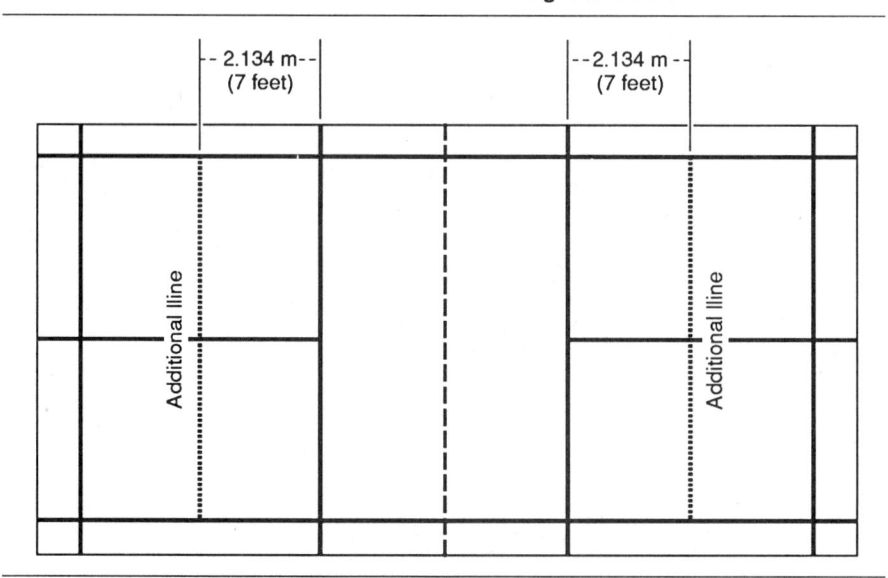

LAW	SEMI-AMBULANT	NON-AMBULANT
11.1.3 and 11.1.4	No Change	As some medical conditions which render a player and "Non-Ambulant" may also positively preclude compliance; these Laws to be deleted in entirely.

11.1.2   The wording of this Law to be extended so as to require every part of the server's and receiver's "mechanical aid" or "support" that is in contact with the surface of the court also to be within the appropriate service court and in a stationary position until the service is delivered. The word "diagonally" to be deleted.

12   *Singles Play*

Shaded area indicates extent of court. As only ONE service court exists at each end, references to 'Left' and 'Right' and 'alternate service court' do not apply.

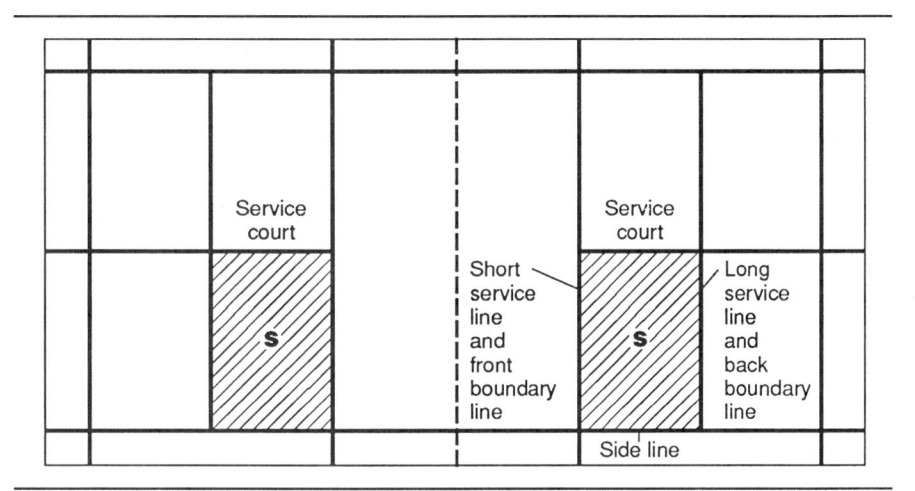

13   *Doubles Play*
Shaded area indicates extent of court.

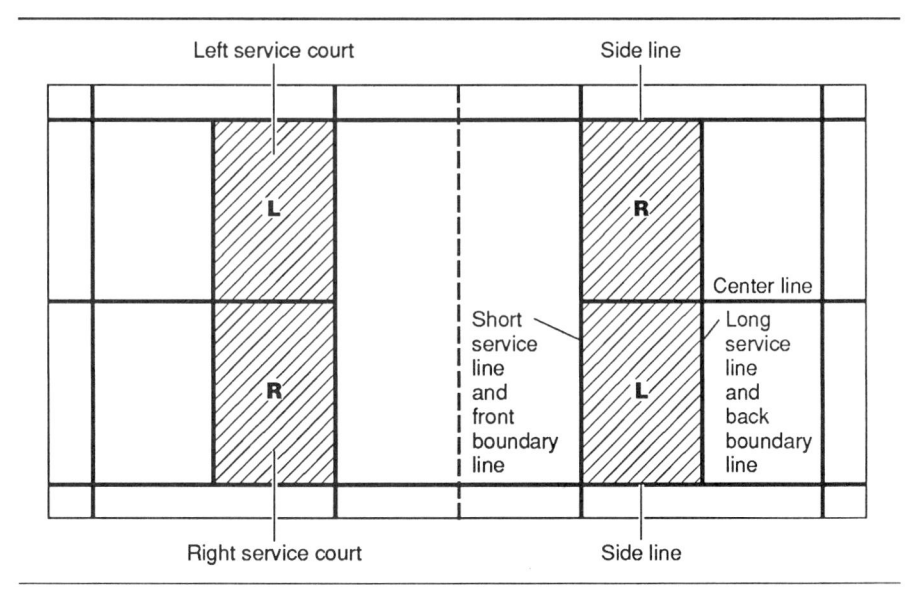

Players must serve from and receive within the same service courts, as adopted at the beginning of a game, throughout that game.

When the service is not returned or a "fault" is made by the receiving side, and the serving side thereby scores a point:

the service passes to the other player of the serving side and is delivered from the other service court and continues to alternate thus as long as the serving side continues to score.

15.4.5 The wording of this Law to be extended so as to make it a "fault" if the player or his "mechanical aid" or "support" touches the shuttle.

All other laws

To remain unchanged for all classifications. (This includes Law 4 with the pace of the shuttle being measured against the length of a standard court by an able-bodied or ambulant player. A shuttle passing this test is suitable for play by all.)

RECOMMENDATIONS TO COURT OFFICIALS

1. INTRODUCTION

1.1 The Recommendations to Court Officials are issued by the IBF in its desire to standardize the control of the game in all countries and in accordance with its Rules.

1.2 The purpose of these Recommendations is to advise Umpires how to control a match firmly and with fairness, without being officious, while ensuring that the Laws of the Game are observed. These Recommendations also give guidance to Service Judges and Line Judges as to how to carry out their duties.

1.3 All court officials should remember that the game is for the players.

2. OFFICIALS AND THEIR DECISIONS

2.1 The Umpire reports to and acts under the authority of the Referee (or the responsible official, in the absence of a Referee).

2.2 A Service Judge is normally appointed by the Referee but can be removed by the Umpire in consultation with the Referee.

2.3 Line Judges are normally appointed by the Referee but a Line Judge can be removed by the Umpire in consultation with the Referee.

2.4 An official's decision is final on all points of fact for which that official is responsible.

2.5 When another official is unsighted, the Umpire makes the decision. When no decision can be given, a "let" is called.

3. RECOMMENDATIONS TO UMPIRES

3.1 Before the match, the Umpire shall:

    3.1.1   obtain the scorepad from the referee;
    3.1.2   ensure that any scoring device to be used is working;
    3.1.3   see that the posts are on the lines, or that the tapes are correctly placed;

	3.1.4	check the net for the height and ensure that there are not gaps between the ends of the net and the net posts;
	3.1.5	ascertain whether there are any by-laws regarding the shuttle hitting an obstruction;
	3.1.6	ensure that the Service Judge and Line Judges know their duties and that they are correctly placed (sections 5 and 6);
	3.1.7	ensure that a sufficient quantity of tested shuttles (Law 4) are readily available for the match in order to avoid delays during play; and
	3.1.8	inform the Referee or appropriate official of any violations of the Tournament Regulations concerning advertising or colored clothing.
3.2	To start the match, the Umpire shall:	
	3.2.1	ensure that the toss is fairly carried out, and that the winning side and the losing side exercise their choice correctly (Law 8);
	3.2.2	note, in the case of doubles, the names of the players starting in the right service court. (Similar notes must be made at the start of each game.) This enables a check to be made at any time to see if the players are in the correct service court. If during the game a player commits a service court error unnoticed, so that the players have to stay wrong, change the note accordingly; and
	3.2.3	(In a tournament) announce the match by calling "Ladies and Gentlemen," "this is the semi-final (or final) of the Men's singles (or, etc.) between .... and ...." "On my right X; and on my left Y" (pointing to right and left as this is said) "X to serve; Y to receive."

or

(In a team event)
"This is the first singles (or, etc.) of the (*e.g.*) Thomas Cup tie between A and B (country names)". "On my right A is represented by X; and on my left B is represented by Y" (pointing to right and left as this is said). "A to serve; love all; play".

(Refer thereafter only to teams, *i.e.*, A and B, rather than players, X and Y).

In Doubles, identify server and receiver by announcing "On my right A is represented by W and X; and on my left B is represented by Y and Z. A to serve; X to Y; love all; play"

3.3	During the match the Umpire shall record and call the score.		
	3.3.1	Always call the server's score first.
	3.3.2	In singles, when a player loses his service, call "Service over" followed by the score in favor of the new server.

3.3.3 In doubles, at the beginning of a game call the score only, and continue to do so as long as the first player serves. When the right to serve is lost call "Service over" followed by the score in favor of the new server. When the first server loses his right to serve, call the score followed by: "Second server."

Continue this as long as the second player serves. When a side loses the right to serve call: "Service over" followed by the score in favor of the new server.

3.3.4 When a side reaches 14, or in the case of Ladies' singles 10, call on the first occasion only in each game. "Game point" or "Match point" when applicable.

If a further game or match point occurs after setting, call it again on the first occasion. "Game point" where applicable should always immediately follow the server's score and precede the receiver's score.

3.3.5 When appropriate, ask the relevant player (side): "Are you setting?" and if the answer if affirmative, call: "Setting _____ points; love-all" (and "second server," if appropriate) or, if the answer is negative, call: "Game not set."

3.3.6 At the end of every game, "game" must always be called immediately after the conclusive rally has ended, regardless of applause. Where appropriate, this constitutes the start of any interval allowed under Law 18.2.

After each game, call:
"Game won by _____ [name(s) of player(s), or team (in a team event)].....[score],"
or if that game wins the match, call:
"Match won by _____ [name(s) of player(s), or team (in a team event)], ...[scores]."

3.3.7 To start the second game, call: "Second Game, love all, play."

3.3.8 If there is to be a third game, call: "One game all" immediately after the call in Recommendation 3.3.6.

If a five minute interval is being claimed, call: "A five minute interval has been claimed."

After three minutes have elapsed, call: "[Court_____] (if appropriate), two minutes remaining." Repeat the call.

After four minutes have elapsed, call: "[Court_____] (if appropriate), one minute remaining." Repeat the call.

To start the third game, call: "Final game; love all; play."

3.3.9 In the third game, or in a one game match, call the score followed by "Change ends" when the leading score reaches 6 or 8, as appropriate (Law 10.1.3).

Once the players have changed ends the score should be repeated, followed by "play."

APPENDIX A 133

- 3.3.10 At the end of the match immediately take the completed scorepad to the Referee.
- 3.4 If a Service Judge is appointed, the Umpire shall especially watch the receiver.
- 3.5 The Umpire should always look to the Line Judge(s) when the shuttle lands close to a line, and always when the shuttle lands out, however far. The Line Judge is entirely responsible for the decision.
- 3.6 During the match the Umpire shall:
  - 3.6.1 if possible, keep aware of the status of any scoring device; and
  - 3.6.2 when the shuttle falls outside a line for which the Umpire is responsible in the absence of a Line Judge, or if the Line Judge is unsighted, call: "Out" before calling the score.
- 3.7 During the match the Umpire shall use the standard vocabulary in Appendix 4 of the Laws of Badminton.
- 3.8 During the match the following situations should be watched for and dealt with as detailed.
  - 3.8.1 A player sliding under the net or throwing a racket into the opponent's court should be faulted under Law 15.6.2.
  - 3.8.2 A player shouting to a partner who is about to hit the shuttle should not necessarily be regarded as distracting his opponent. Calling "no shot," "fault," etc. should be considered a distraction.
  - 3.8.3 Coaching during a match from off court should be prevented. If this cannot be controlled by the Umpire, the Referee should be informed immediately.
  - 3.8.4 Players going off court to wipe their hands, etc. If play is not held up, this is acceptable, but if one side is ready to play, the offending side may have to be reminded that leaving the court needs the Umpire's permission (Law 18.5.2), and if necessary Law 18.8 should be applied.
  - 3.8.5 Changing the shuttle during the match should not be unfair. If both sides agree to the change, there should be no objection by the Umpire. If only one side wishes to change the shuttle, the Umpire should make the decision, testing the shuttle if necessary.
  - 3.8.6 Law 15.8. A double hit by one player with one stroke is not a "fault."
- 3.9 Ensure that players do not leave the court without the Umpire's permission.
- 3.10 Injury or sickness during a match must be handled carefully and flexibly. The Umpire must determine the severity of the problem as quickly as possible. Normally, the only people that should be allowed on court are a doctor or paramedical, and the Referee.

The opposing side must not be put at a disadvantage and Laws 11.1.1 and 18.4 should be applied appropriately.

3.11 If play has to be suspended, call "Play is suspended" and record the score, server, receiver, correct service court and ends.

When play resumes call "Are you ready," call the score (and, if appropriate "first server") and "play."

3.12 A shuttle whose speed has been interfered with should be discarded.

3.13 Misconduct

    3.13.1 Record and report to the Referee any incidents of misconduct and the action taken.

    3.13.2 If Law 18.8 is to be applied, call "come here please" to the offending player, and call "____ (name of player), warning for misconduct" or ____ (name of player), fault for misconduct." at the same time raising the right hand above your head.

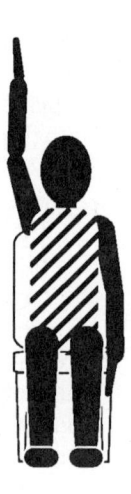

4. GENERAL ADVICE ON UMPIRING

This section gives general advice which should be followed.

4.1 Know and understand the "Laws of Badminton."

4.2 Call promptly and with authority, but, if a mistake is made, admit it, apologize and correct it.

4.3 All announcements and calling of the score must be done distinctly and loudly enough to be heard clearly by players and spectators.

4.4 When a doubt arises in your mind as to whether an infringement of the Laws has occurred or not, "fault" should not be called and the game allowed to proceed.

4.5 Never ask spectators nor be influenced by their remarks.

APPENDIX A 135

4.6 Motivate your other Court Officials, e.g., by discreetly acknowledging the decisions of the Line Judges and establishing a working relationship with them.

5. INSTRUCTIONS TO SERVICE JUDGES

5.1 The Service Judge shall sit on a low chair by the post, preferably opposite the Umpire.

5.2 The Service Judge is responsible for judging that the server delivers a correct service (Law 11.1). If not, call "fault" loudly and use the approved hand signal to indicate the type of infringement.

5.3 The approved hand signals are:

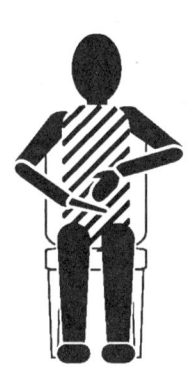

Law 11.1.3

The initial point of contact with the shuttle not on the base of the shuttle.

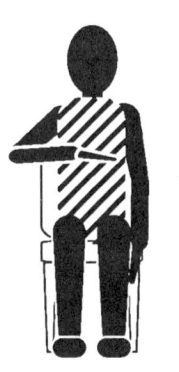

Law 11.1.3

Any part of the shuttle at the instant of being struck higher than the server's waist.

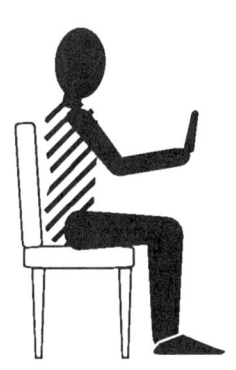

Law 11.1.4

At the instant of the shuttle being hit, the shaft of the racket not pointing in a downward direction to such an extent that the whole of the head of the racket is discernibly below the whole of the server's hand holding the racket.

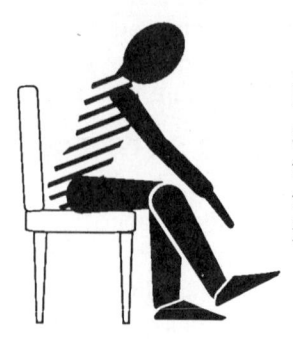

Law 11.1.2

Some part of both feet not in the service court and in a stationary position until the service is delivered.

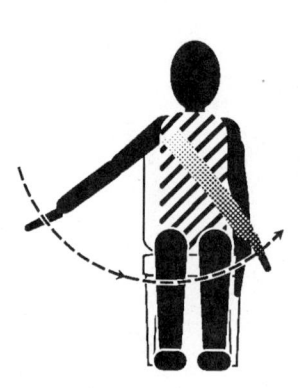

Laws 11.1.1, 11.2 and 11.1.5

Undue delay to the delivery of the service. Once the players have taken their positions the first foward movement of the server's racket is the start of the service. The movement must continue forward.

5.4 The Umpire may arrange with the Service Judge any extra duties to be undertaken, provided that the players are so advised.

6. INSTRUCTIONS TO LINE JUDGES

6.1 Line Judges should be sited on chairs in prolongation of their lines at the ends and sides of the court and preferably at the side opposite to the Umpire. (See diagram C).

6.2 A Line Judge is entirely responsible for the line(s) assigned. If the shuttle lands out, no matter how far, call "Out" promptly in a clear voice, loud enough to be heard by the players and the spectators and, at the same time, signal by extending both arms horizontally so that the Umpire can see clearly.

If the shuttle falls in, the Line Judge shall say nothing, but point to the line with the right hand.

6.3 If unsighted, inform the Umpire immediately by putting both hands up to cover the eyes.

6.4 Do not call or signal until the shuttle has touched the floor.

6.5 Calls should always be made, and no anticipation made of Umpiring decisions, e.g. that the shuttle hit a player.

APPENDIX A

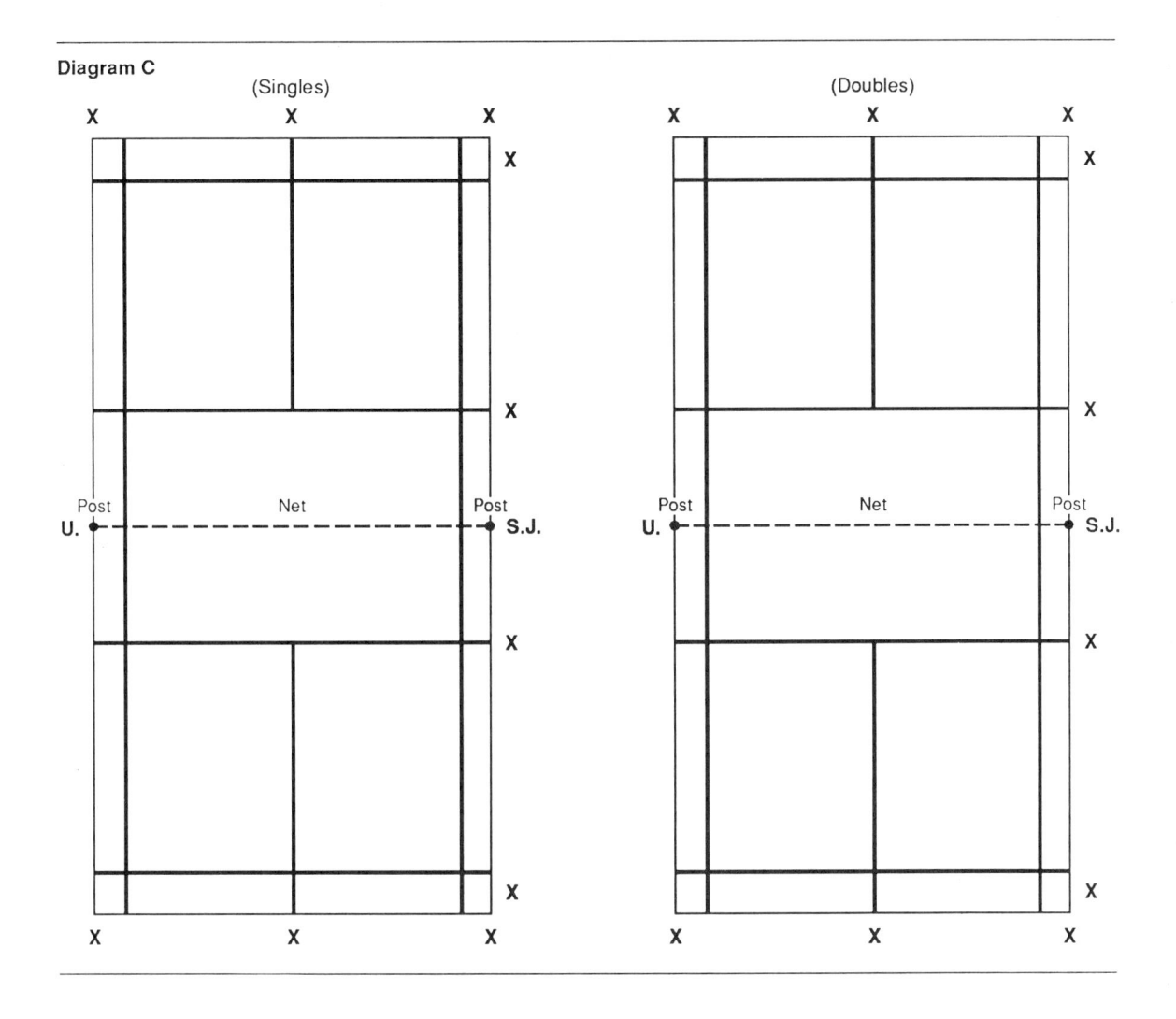

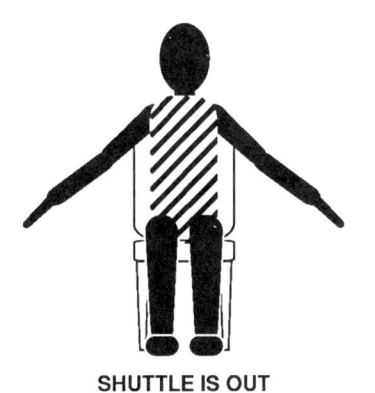

Diagram C

(Singles)

(Doubles)

SHUTTLE IS OUT

Signals for Line Judges

If the shuttle lands out, no matter how far, call "out" promptly in a clear voice, loud enough to be heard by the players and the spectators and, at the same time, signal by extending both arms horizontally so that the Umpire can see clearly.

SHUTTLE IS IN

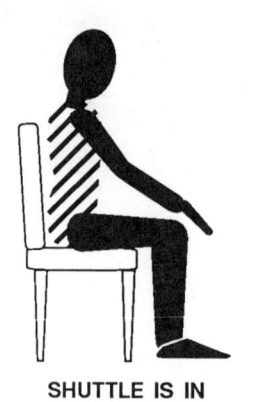

If the shuttle falls "in", say nothing, but point to the line with your right hand.

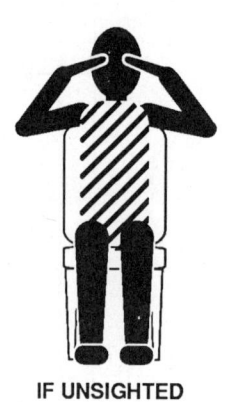

IF UNSIGHTED

If unsighted, inform the Umpire immediately by holding your hands to cover your eyes.

APPENDIX B

The United States Badminton Association

The National Governing Body of U.S. Badminton*

Function

The United States Badminton Association is the official association of organized badminton in the United States, recognized as the National Governing Body (NGB) by both the United States Olympic Committee (USOC) and the International Badminton Federation (IBF). As such, it promulgates to its members not only the official rules of play, as laid down by the IBF, but also other pertinent information from both the IBF and USOC for the benefit of USBA members and organizations.

Activities Sponsored

a. All tournaments are conducted under standard regulations, and must receive sanctions to be held, thus insuring proper ranking and operation for the benefit of the contestants.
b. Amateur standards have been established to preserve the proper distinction between amateurs and professionals.
c. National rules for umpiring are controlled by a national Rules Committee, thus insuring a uniform code for all playing areas.
d. Juniors have special development activities which include intersectional, national and international tournaments all under programs which steadily improve each year.
e. Many sectional adult and senior tournaments are held during the year plus one national tournament for both groups. These are highly competitive events which are generally concluded with a relaxing social event.
f. Individuals and teams of men and women of top ranking caliber are selected for national and international play and exhibitions.

Publication

Badminton USA, a national publication, is published under the guidance and backing of the national association, providing the official vehicle for distribution of information on all phases of badminton, much of which is not available from any other source.

---

*Excerpted and reprinted from *Official Rules of Play*, © 1987, p. 627, with permission from the United States Badminton Association.

Membership

For your pleasure or that of your group, whether interested in competition or not, a membership in the USBA at nominal rates, will bring you greater knowledge of the game and the advantages listed above. If you are interested in club or individual membership, the National Office will furnish you the necessary forms or information on request.

APPENDIX C

Tournament Operation*

1. A tournament worth holding deserves good planning. Confusion in management results in confused contestants and many may not want to play again.
2. Where the time element for completion of certain rounds is important, be strict in the times for the matches, always recognizing that the players are human. Don't browbeat them or make it a military split second job.
3. Special rules specific to individual sites should be properly posted and announced for complete understanding of all participants.
4. Seek help in establishing seeding and making the draw from persons in nearby clubs or associations who have experience in these areas. Additionally, the National Office personnel will be pleased to assist.
5. USBA has an equipment testing program to determine the adequacy of equipment utilized during sanctioned tournaments.
6. Try to use umpires on at least all rounds from the semifinals on but select as qualified a group as possible. When holding Junior events it is wise to umpire each match.
7. National rules for the United States have rest periods of 5 minutes between the second and third game of all events, if any one player requests it. A five-minute rest period between the second and third games in all Junior events is mandatory. Additionally, the tournament director may authorize a 5 minute rest period after the first game. If he does allow this rest period, it should be made known in special instructions.
8. Except for these rest periods, play is continuous. If accidents occur, the umpire (or tournament referee if there is no umpire on the match) may make special rulings to cover the situation. Towel wiping, drinking water and the like are to be permitted in the confines of the court only and are not to be used for stalling.

Match Scheduling

The USBA Match Scheduling System is a procedure for "programming" a tournament so that each match in each event is scheduled at a definite time on a specific court. Control is exercised through the use of master schedules by the director of play and individual cards for each player. Each separate match is numbered which permits precise scheduling.

Details in the use of the USBA Match Scheduling System may be secured from the USBA National Office.

Due to the many rules on drug testing, it suffices to say here that sooner or later all international and national athletes will be subject to drug testing. The testing will be at unannounced times with individuals chosen at random.

---

*Excerpted and reprinted from *Official Rules of Play*, © 1987, pps. 10–20, with permission from the United States Badminton Association.

Results will be confidential. Persons using drugs will be appropriately disciplined. Athletes are cautioned that some of the over-the-counter drugs or prescriptions may show up in the testing process so competitors should let officials know about all medications.

Detailed rules on drug testing are available at the National Office for those interested.

The Draw

1. The draw for International Championships and other international events shall be made in the manner set out below and no dummy entry is permitted. (National and local tourneys should also conform to these provisions).
2. The tournament committee or referee shall not—except according to Regulation 6 below—permit any alteration to the published draw of any of these events except in the following circumstances:
   a. the original player/pair is prevented from competing through illness, injury, or other unavoidable hindrance;
   b. the substitute player/pair would not have attained a seeded place higher than the original player/pair.
3. Substitution in singles is then permitted:
   a. when entries are limited solely by nomination from national associations,
   b. to enable a foreign player to replace a player from the same association provided that the original player does not participate in the tournament.
4. Substitution is then permitted:
   a. to enable a doubles pair to have a substitute partner provided the constitution of no other doubles pair is affected except if substitutes be permitted in two doubles pairings the remaining players shall be permitted to partner with each other;
   b. if one of the original pairs has drawn a bye, that place in the draw shall be filled by the new pairing otherwise the place shall be drawn by lot.
5. A player shall compete once only in the same event at any tournament.
6. Qualifying Rounds

   Where entries exceed the required places in the main competition draw, the organizers are recommended to play qualifying rounds under the supervision of the tournament committee or referee as follows:

   a. the players or pairs not directly in the main competition shall play for a limited number of places fixed by the organizers;
   b. it is recommended that the main draw does not include more than one qualifier for eight places;
   c. where players or pairs withdraw their entry from the main competition before the qualifying rounds have started, the organizers may fill the vacancies from the entries in these qualifying rounds;
   d. the players to fill vacancies in the main competition shall beforehand be selected in order of strength and placed in the draw by lot.
   e. if more players or pairs enter the competition than the organizers can

accept even in the qualifying rounds then these players/pairs shall beforehand be selected in order of strength and shall, in case of vacancies, be put into the qualifying rounds and placed in the draw by lot.

7. Regulations for Making the Draw

The draw shall be conducted as follows:

When the number of playing units is 4, 8, 16, 32, 64, or any higher power of 2, they shall meet in pairs in the order drawn, as in the following diagram:

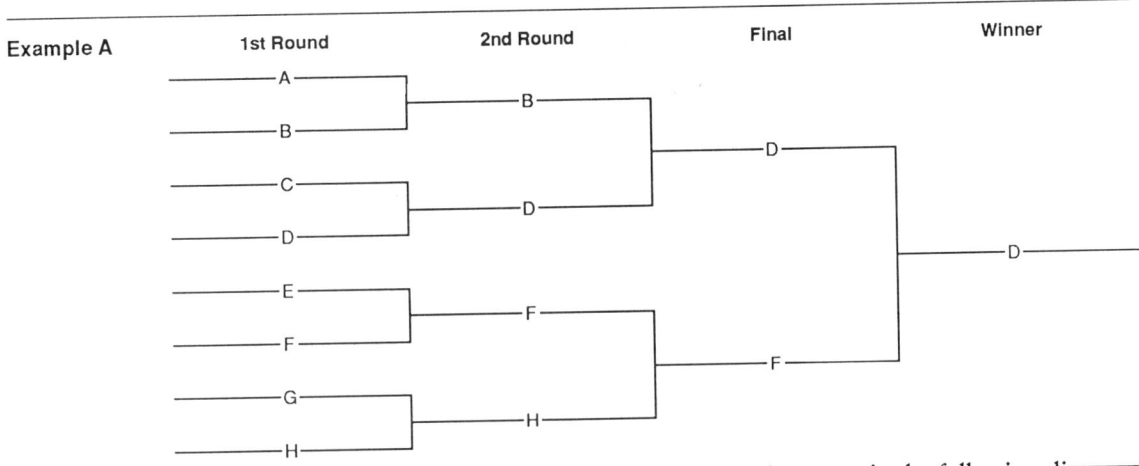

Example A

```
          1st Round      2nd Round       Final        Winner
            ─A─
               ├──B──┐
            ─B─      │
                     ├──D──┐
            ─C─      │     │
               ├──D──┘     │
            ─D─            ├──D──┐
                           │     │
            ─E─            │     │
               ├──F──┐     │     │
            ─F─      │     │     ├──D──
                     ├──F──┘     │
            ─G─      │           │
               ├──H──┘           │
            ─H─                  │
```

When the number of playing units is not a power of 2, there shall be byes in the first round. The number of byes shall be equal to the difference between the next highest power of 2 and the number of playing units. The byes, if even in number, shall be divided, as the names are drawn in equal proportions at the top and bottom of the list, above and below the pairs; if uneven in number, there shall be one more bye at the bottom than at the top.

Example: With 19 playing units there will be 32 - 19 = 13 byes, 6 at the top and 7 at the bottom of the list, and 3 matches in the first round, 8 in the second, 4 in the third, etc.

Example: With 9 playing units there will be 16 - 9 = 7 byes, 3 at the top, and 4 at the bottom, and one match in the first round thus:

Example B

```
       1st Round    2nd Round   3rd Round     Final     Winner
         Bye
                  ─── A ───┐
         Bye                ├── B ──┐
                  ─── B ───┘        │
         Bye                         ├── B ──┐
                  ─── C ───┐        │       │
          ─D─              ├── D ──┘        │
             ├             │                 │
          ─E─   ─── D ───┘                  ├── B ──
         Bye                                 │
                  ─── F ───┐                 │
         Bye                ├── G ──┐        │
                  ─── G ───┘        │       │
         Bye                         ├── G ──┘
                  ─── H ───┐        │
         Bye                ├── I ──┘
                  ─── I ───┘
```

With 5 playing units there will be 1 bye at the top and 2 byes at the bottom.
With 6, 1 bye at the top, and 1 bye at the bottom.
With 7, 1 bye at the bottom.
With 8, no byes.
With 9, 3 byes at the top, and 4 byes at the bottom.
With 10, 3 byes at the top, and 3 byes at the bottom.
With 11, 2 byes at the top, and 3 byes at the bottom.
With 12, 2 byes at the top, and 2 byes at the bottom.
With 13, 1 bye at the top, and 2 byes at the bottom.
With 14, 1 bye at the top, and 1 bye at the bottom.
With 15, 1 bye at the bottom.
With 16, no byes.
And so on with larger numbers in like manner.

8. Instead of the method described in Regulation 4, the draw can be made so that the byes due are distributed as nearly as possible equally in the four quarters and in the following manner:

   a. If the total number of byes exceeds the power of 4 immediately below that number, then the first additional bye shall be placed in the fourth quarter, the second in the first quarter, and the third in the third quarter.
   b. The byes in the first and second quarters shall be placed all at the top of those quarters, and the byes in the third and fourth quarters all at the bottom of those quarters. (See example "C")

Regulations for Seeding the Draw

NOTE: For USBA Tournaments other than the Open Amateur Championships the following modifications for the Seed have been approved: In case of an entry of 12 or more, but less than 16, there may be two entries placed in addition to the two seeded entries; and in the case of an entry of 24 or more, but less than 32 entries, there may be two entries placed in addition to the four seeded.

1. The seeded entries shall be drawn as follows:

   a. If two are to be seeded, numbers 1 and 2 shall be drawn by lot; the first drawn shall be placed at the top of the upper half and the second at the bottom of the lower half.
   b. If four are to be seeded, numbers 1, 2, 3, and 4 shall be placed as above; numbers 3 and 4 shall be drawn by lot and the first drawn shall be placed at the top of the second quarter; the second shall be placed at the bottom of third quarter.
   c. If eight are to be seeded, numbers 1, 2, 3, and 4 shall be placed as above; the remainder shall be drawn by lot and placed in the upper half, at the top of the eighths not already occupied and in the lower half, at the bottom of the eighths not already occupied. (Example B.)

2. Any two entries from any country which shall be seeded shall be drawn in separate halves of the draw, and any three or four entries from any one country which shall be seeded shall be drawn in separate quarters of the draw. NOTE: In the United States, Regions should be considered as countries in this regard. Players from the same Region should not play each other in the first round in singles, or in doubles if both players on

Example C: Seeded draw

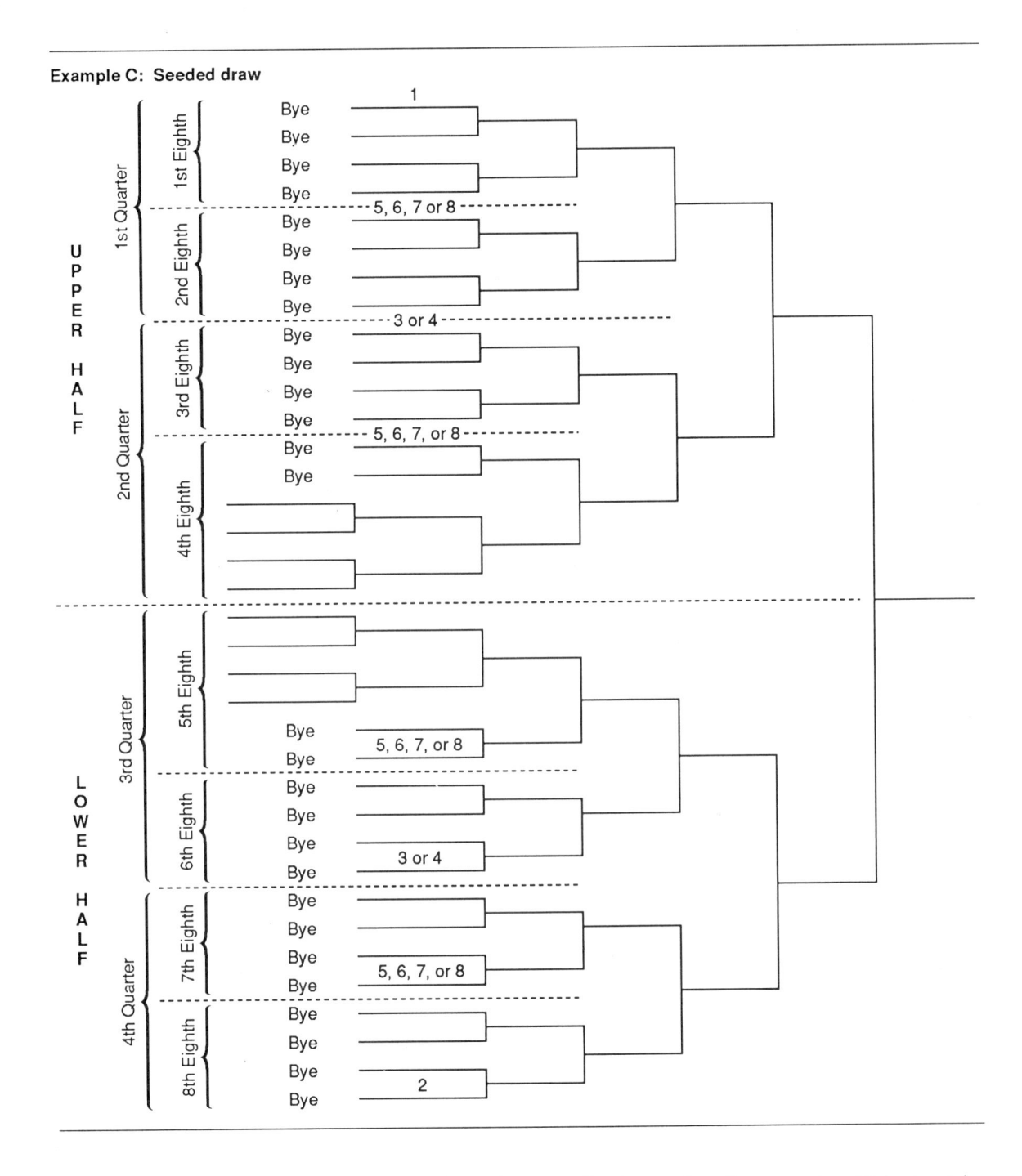

[Bracket diagram showing a seeded draw for a 64-position tournament bracket:

UPPER HALF
- 1st Quarter
  - 1st Eighth: Bye, Bye, Bye, Bye — seed 1
  - 2nd Eighth: Bye, Bye, Bye, Bye — 5, 6, 7 or 8
- 2nd Quarter
  - 3rd Eighth: Bye, Bye, Bye, Bye — 3 or 4
  - 4th Eighth: Bye, Bye — 5, 6, 7, or 8

LOWER HALF
- 3rd Quarter
  - 5th Eighth
  - 6th Eighth: Bye, Bye, Bye, Bye — 5, 6, 7, or 8
- 4th Quarter
  - 7th Eighth: Bye, Bye, Bye, Bye — 3 or 4
  - 8th Eighth: Bye, Bye, Bye, Bye — 5, 6, 7, or 8 / seed 2]

each team are from the same Region, unless there are insufficient entries to do otherwise.

3. In addition to the seeded entries, in the case of only two entries from any one country, they shall be drawn in separate halves of the draw, and not less than the four best entries from one country, but not more than eight, shall be drawn in separate quarters or eighths as the case may be. NOTE: Again treat states or regions in the United States as countries in this manner.

Example D: Placing byes

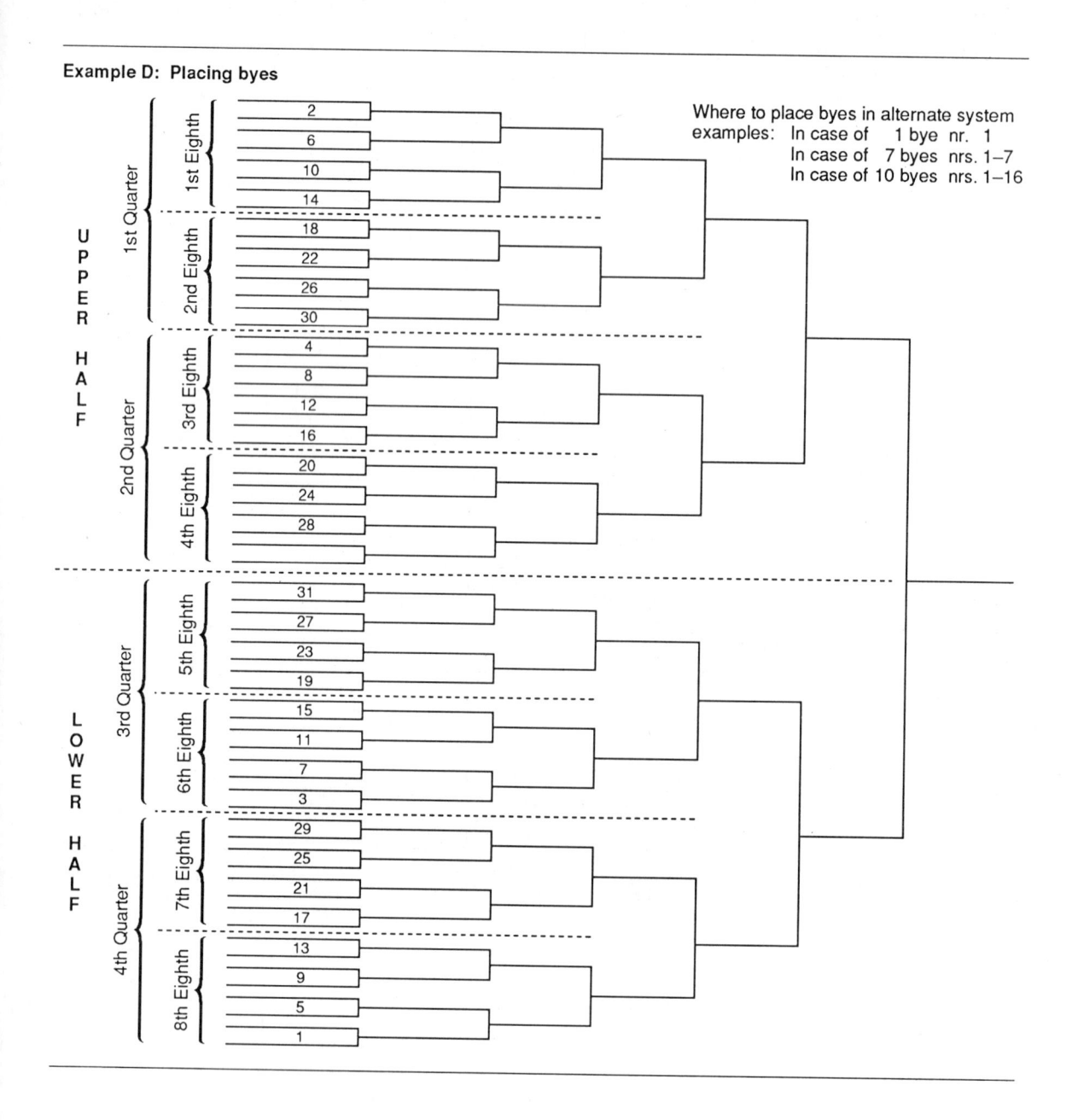

Where to place byes in alternate system examples:
In case of 1 bye nr. 1
In case of 7 byes nrs. 1–7
In case of 10 byes nrs. 1–16

UPPER HALF

1st Quarter
- 1st Eighth: 2, 6, 10, 14
- 2nd Eighth: 18, 22, 26, 30

2nd Quarter
- 3rd Eighth: 4, 8, 12, 16
- 4th Eighth: 20, 24, 28

LOWER HALF

3rd Quarter
- 5th Eighth: 31, 27, 23, 19
- 6th Eighth: 15, 11, 7, 3

4th Quarter
- 7th Eighth: 29, 25, 21, 17
- 8th Eighth: 13, 9, 5, 1

Some Hints on Doing the Draw

Tournament secretaries and others frequently find difficulty in quickly producing a correct draw for events with uneven numbers of entrants, particularly insofar as the placing of byes and seeded entrants is concerned. Certainly, it is not an easy matter, and it is hoped that the following table will be helpful.

The most satisfactory method of producing the draw is on a typewriter when several carbon copies can be made.

Firstly, type in column form on plain paper numbers from 1, 2, 3, downwards, down to the total number of entrants.

Secondly, insert to the right of the typed number, where it is appropriate, the word "bye" and an asterisk in the case of a seeded position. These places in the draw can be ascertained from the following table which gives the correct information for every number of entries from 16 to 64. In the case of events containing less than 16 entrants there should be little difficulty, and beyond 64 (which is rare) the principle will be identical.

Thirdly, type in the players' names in their appropriate place as they are drawn.

It will be found that, by having followed the instructions in the table below, the brackets for the different rounds can be inserted in ink.

It is to be noted that the regulations do not permit the seeding of more than two entrants when there are less than 16 players or pairs, and of more than four entrants where the total is less than 32. Eight seeded entrants is the maximum allowed.

Example E: Byes and Seeding Positions in the Draw

Number of Entries	Placing of Byes		Seeded Positions						
	Top	Bottom	1–2	5–8	3–4	5–8	5–8	3–4	1–2
									5–8
16	–	–	1	–	5	–	–	12	–	16
17	1–7	10–17	1	–	5	–	–	13	–	17
18	1–7	12–18	1	–	5	–	–	14	–	18
19	1–6	13–19	1	–	5	–	–	15	–	19
20	1–6	15–20	1	–	5	–	–	16	–	20
21	1–5	16–21	1	–	5	–	–	17	–	21
22	1–5	18–22	1	–	5	–	–	18	–	22
23	1–4	19–23	1	–	5	–	–	19	–	23
24	1–4	21–24	1	–	5	–	–	20	–	24
25	1–3	22–25	1	–	6	–	–	21	–	25
26	1–3	24–26	1	–	6	–	–	21	–	26
27	1–2	25–27	1	–	7	–	–	22	–	27
28	1–2	27–28	1	–	7	–	–	22	–	28
29	1	28–29	1	–	8	–	–	23	–	29
30	1	30	1	–	8	–	–	23	–	30
31	–	31	1	–	9	–	–	24	–	31
32	–	–	1	5	9	13	20	24	28	32
33	1–15	18–33	1	5	9	13	21	25	29	33
34	1–15	20–34	1	5	9	13	22	26	30	34

continued

Example E: Byes and Seeding Positions in the Draw (continued)

Number of Entries	Placing of Byes Top	Placing of Byes Bottom	1–2	Seeded Positions 5–8	Seeded Positions 3–4	Seeded Positions 5–8	Seeded Positions 5–8	Seeded Positions 3–4	Seeded Positions 5–8	1–2
35	1–14	21–35	1	5	9	13	23	27	31	35
36	1–14	23–36	1	5	9	13	24	28	32	36
37	1–13	24–37	1	5	9	13	25	29	33	37
38	1–13	26–38	1	5	9	13	26	30	34	38
39	1–12	27–39	1	5	9	13	27	31	35	39
40	1–12	29–40	1	5	9	13	28	32	36	40
41	1–11	30–41	1	5	9	14	29	33	37	41
42	1–11	32–42	1	5	9	14	29	34	38	42
43	1–10	33–43	1	5	9	15	30	35	39	43
44	1–10	35–44	1	5	9	15	30	36	40	44
45	1–9	36–45	1	5	9	16	31	37	41	45
46	1–9	38–46	1	5	9	16	31	38	42	46
47	1–8	39–47	1	5	9	17	32	39	43	47
48	1–8	41–48	1	5	9	17	32	40	44	48
49	1–7	42–49	1	5	10	18	33	41	45	49
50	1–7	44–50	1	5	10	18	33	41	46	50
51	1–6	45–51	1	5	11	19	34	42	47	51
52	1–6	47–52	1	5	11	19	34	42	48	52
53	1–5	48–53	1	5	12	20	35	43	49	53
54	1–5	50–54	1	5	12	20	35	43	50	54
55	1–4	51–55	1	5	13	21	36	44	51	55
56	1–4	53–56	1	5	13	21	36	44	52	56
57	1–3	54–57	1	6	14	22	37	45	53	57
58	1–3	56–58	1	6	14	22	37	45	53	58
59	1–2	57–59	1	7	15	23	38	46	54	59
60	1–2	59–60	1	7	15	23	38	46	54	60
61	1	60-61	1	8	16	24	39	47	55	61
62	1	62	1	8	16	24	39	47	55	62
63	–	63	1	9	17	25	40	48	56	63
64	–	–	1	9	17	25	40	48	56	64

APPENDIX D

Badminton Clubs in the United States

AK	Anchorage Badminton Club	700 W. 58th Ave. Unit D, Anchorage, AK 99518	907/563-6112
AZ	Belvedere Country Club	Route 18, Box 114, Hot Springs, AZ 71901	501/623-9227
CA	Southern California B. A.	P. O. Box 1435, Culver City, CA 90232	213/439-9433
CA	University of California-Davis	140 Recreation Hall Intramural Office, Davis, CA 95616	916/752-3500
CA	Peninsula Badminton Club	757-A Calderon Ave., Mountain View, CA 94041	415/961-3865
CA	Mar Vista Badminton Club	3269 Coolidge Ave. Los Angeles, CA 90066	213/398-6837
CA	Manhattan Beach B. C.	516 18th Street P.O. Box 3339, Manhattan Beach, CA 90266	213/545-9052
CA	San Diego Badminton Club	6135 Syracuse Lane, San Diego, CA 92122	619/455-9331
CA	Castilleja School	1310 Bryant Street, Palo Alto, CA 94301	415/366-4929
CA	Northern California B. A.	C/O Len Hill 757-A Calderon, Mountain View, CA 94041	
CA	Long Beach Badminton Club	2435 E. Broadway, Long Beach, CA 90803	213/439-9433
CA	Riverside Badminton Club	P. O. Box 7473, Riverside, CA 92503	714/351-1104
CA	Rolm-AM IBM Company	4900 Old Ironside Drive M/S 459, Santa Clara, CA 95054	408/986-4244
CA	Chandler School	1005 Armada Dr., Pasadena, CA 91001	818/791-9137
CA	Claremont Colleges B. C.	Summer Hall #201 Pomona College, Claremont, CA 91711	714/621-8328
CA	State Capitol Badminton Club	P. O. Box 2089, Sacramento, CA 95810	916/636-4246
CA	UCLA Badminton Club	John Wooden Center, U.C.L.A., CA 90024	213/825-3701
CA	East Los Angeles B. C.	1301 Brooklyn Ave. Women's P.E., Monterey Park, CA 91754	213/265-8919
CA	Sunnyvale Badminton Club	839 Pagoda Tree Court, Sunnyvale, CA 94086	408/735-8484
CO	Colorado Badminton Association	85 Southmoor Drive, Denver, CO 80220	303/333-5678
CO	Elite Rocky Mountain B. C.	826 London Green Way, Colorado Springs, CO 80906	303/579-0746
CT	Greenwich Boys & Girls Club	4 Horseneck Lane, Greenwich, CT 06830	203/869-3224
CT	Greenwich Badminton Club	39 Jones Park, Riverside, CT 06878	203/637-2623
CT	Greenwich High School	12 N. Sound Beach Ave., Riverside, CT 06878	
CT	Sport System Inc.	1360 Galloping Hill Rd., Fairfield, CT 06430	203/254-0918
CT	Greenwich YWCA	259 E. Putman Ave., Greenwich, CT 06830	203/869-6501
CT	New Haven Badminton Club	2195 Shepard Ave., New Haven, CT 06518	
CT	Brunswick School	100 Maher Ave., Greenwich, CT 06830	
CT	Greenwich Academy	200 N. Maple Ave., Greenwich, CT 06830	
CT	Connecticut Badminton Assoc.	12 Byron Drive, Granby, CT 06035	203/653-7398
DC	District of Columbia Assoc.	4547 Grant Rd., N.W., Washington, DC 20016	202/686-5026
DC	Pentagon Officers Athlete Club	Dept. of the Army, The Pentagon, Room BG 877, Washington, DC 20310-0007	703/521-5020
DE	Delaware State Association	10 Forest Ave., Claymont, DE 19703	
FL	Florida State Association	7242 Lochness Dr., Miami Lakes, FL 33014	
FL	Miami Badminton Club	2312 S.W. 16th Terrace, Miami, FL 33145	305/856-9671
FL	Univeristy Of Florida B. C.	208 Florida Gym, Univ. of Florida, Gainesville, FL 32611	904/392-0581
GA	Georgia State University B. C.	Box 189, Georgia State University, Atlanta, GA 30301	404/378-8922

GA	Oxford College of Emory Univ.	Oxford, GA 30267	404/784-8350
GA	Spelman Badminton Club	Spelman College, 350 Spelman Lane, S.W., Atlanta, GA 30314-4399	404/681-3643
GA	Georgia State Association	Atlanta Athletic Club, Athletic Club Drive, Duluth, GA 30136	
HI	Hilo Badminton Club	P. O. Box 1533, Hilo, HI 96721	808/959-7829
IL	Rockford Badminton Club	YWCA, 220 S. Madison, Rockford, IL 61108	815/968-9681
IL	Midwest Badminton Association	65 S. Meyer Court, Des Plaines, IL 60016	312/869-9803
IL	University of Chicago B. C.	5125 S. Elllis Ave., Chicago, IL 60615	312/324-8331
IL	Lyons Badminton Club	3406 Hollywood Ave., Brookfield, IL 60513	312/485-6137
LA	New Orleans Badminton Club	4846 Camp Street, New Orleans, LA 70115	
LA	Southern Badminton Association	347 Corinne Circle, Shreveport, LA 71106	
MA	Bird & Bottle Club	Box 61 P, S. Dartmouth, MA 02748	
MA	Maugus Club	40 Abbott Rd., Wellesley Hills, MA 02181	617/235-8151
MA	Massachusetts State Assoc.	4 Mitton Circle, Andover, MA 01810	617/479-2690
MD	Garrison Forest School	Garrison, MD 21055	301/363-8904
MD	Badminton Club of Wash. D.C.	11303 Dewey Road, Silver Spring, MD 20906	301/946-3924
MD	Maryland State Association	127 Willow Bend Dr., Owings Mills, MD 21117	
MD	University of Maryland B. C.	Room 1104, Reckord Armory, College Park, MD 20742-5311	301/454-3124
ME	Maine State B. A.	21 Orchard Street, Portland, ME 04106	207/799-5288
MI	Birmingham Badminton Club	28925 Millbrook Rd., Farmington Hills, MI 48018	313/626-0315
MI	Ann Arbor Badminton Club	3134 Sunnywood, Ann Arbor, MI 48103	313/662-4819
MI	Grosse Pointe Badminton Assoc.	165 Lothrop, Grosse Pointe Farms, MI 48236	
MI	Dearborn Westwood B. C.	2010 Hollywood, Dearborn, MI 48124	313/336-5959
MN	Minneapolis Athletic Club	615 Second Ave. S., Minneapolis, MN 55402	612/339-3655
MN	St. Paul Athletic Club	340 Cedar Street, St. Paul, MN 55101	612/222-3661
MO	St. Louis Badminton Club	11959 Cleychester Dr.,St. Louis, MO 63131	314/966-3595
NC	Duke University	Dept. of Health & Phys. Ed., Durham, NC 27706	
NC	North Carolina State Assoc.	239 Scofield Rd., Charlotte, NC 28209	
NE	Top Flight Badminton Club	501 W. 6th St., Papillon, NE 68046	402/592-7309
NH	Key Hampshire State Assoc.	7 Ledge Circle, Concord, NH 03301	603/225-9658
NJ	New Jersey State Association	42 Roosevelt Ave., Morganville, NJ 07751	201/591-9167
NJ	Mountain Lakes Badminton Club	Route 1, Box 221, Chester, NJ 07930	201/879-5167
NJ	Washiington Township B. C.	252 West Valley Brook Road, Califon, NJ 07830	201/832-5120
NM	Mesilla Valley Badminton Club	1502 N. Tornillo Street, Las Cruces, NM 88001	505/524-4265
NY	New York State Association	Wolfs Hill Rd., Chappaqua, NY 10514	914/238-4947
NY	Metropolitan Badminton Assoc.	500 West 111th Street,#4G, New York, NY 10025	212/866-1162
NY	New York Athletic Club	75 East End Ave., New York, NY 10028	212/249-2396
NY	Northeast Badminton Assoc.	Wolfs Hill Rd., Chappaqua, NY 10514	914/238-4947
NY	Miller Place Badminton Club	P. O. Box 780, Miller Place, NY 11764	516/473-6701
NY	Western New York B. A.	50 Tiberlake Dr., Orchard Park, NY 14127	716/662-0308
NY	Badminton Club of City of N. Y.	50 East 72nd Street Apt. #15A, New York, NY 10021	212/772-1959
NY	New York University	Coles Sports Center, 181 Mercer St., New York, NY 10012	212/998-2033
NY	Columbia U. Badminton Club	Iris Chan Dodge Gym, New York City, NY 10027	212-889-0909
NY	United National B. C.	42nd Street, 1st Ave. Room S-21491, New York, NY 10017	212/963-6256
NY	The Hewitt School	45 E. 75th Street, New York, NY 10021	212/288-1919
NY	Garden City Badminton Club	79 North Street Pauls Rd., Hempstead, NY 11550	516/483-8185

APPENDIX D 151

OH	Shaker Badminton Club	2584 Dartmoor Road, Cleveland Heights, OH 44118	216/932-6306
OH	Ohio State Association	Sinclair Community College, Dayton, OH 45402	
OK	Oklahoma State Association	P. O. Box 1267, Ponca City, OK 74603	
OR	Oregon State Association	2581 Willakenzie #4, Eugene, Or 97401-4812	
OR	Univerity of Orgeon B. C.	EMU Club Sports, EMU Rm 5, Univ. of Oregon, Eugene, OR 97403	503/686-3733
OR	Multnomah Athletic Club	1849 S. W. Salmon Street, Portland, OR 97205	503/223-8740
PA	Mansfield Badminton Club	Mansfield University, Mansfield, PA 16933	717/638-3266
PA	New Philadelphia Regional B. A.	255 F Shawmont, Philadelphia, PA 19128	215/482-7840
PA	Wissahickon Badminton Club	Germantown Cricket Club, Manhaeim & Morris Streets, Philadelphia, PA 19144	215/438-9900
PA	Drexel Varsity Badminton	32nd & Chestnut, Philadelphia, PA 19104	215/895-2982
PA	Pennsylvania Badminton Assoc.	8309 Crittenden Street, Philadelphia, PA 19118	215/247-0490
RI	Rhode Island State B. A.	175 Pequot Trail, East Greenwich, RI 02818	401/732-4368
SC	South Carolina State Assoc.	1400 Devonshire Dr., Columbia, SC 29208	
TX	Texas A & M Badminton Club	Texas A & M Univ., 159 Read Building, College Station, TX 77843-4243	409/260-7982
TX	Texas State Association	2590 Morgan Ave., Corpus Christi, TX 78405	
VA	College of William & Mary	Office of Rec. Sports, Blov Gym, Rm 4, Williamsburg, VA 23185	804/253-4360
VA	Sports Network	8320 Quarry Road, Manassas, VA 22110	703/631-0037
VA	Virginia State Association	3804 N. 18th Street, Arlington, VA 22207	703/243-5464
VA	Rockville Badminton Club	1021 Arlington Blvd., #E422, Arlington, VA 22209	202/328-2797
VT	Vermont State Association	38 Farmview Rd., Williston, VT 05495	802/878-1199
WA	Highline Badminton Club	16815 27th S.W., Seattle, WA 98166	206/242-3885
WI	Univ. of Wisconsin-Madison B. C.	Recreational Sports 2000 Observatory Dr., Madison, WI 53706	608/231-3092
WI	Greater Milwaukee B. C.	21800 Gareth Lane, Brookfield, WI 53005	
WI	Madison Badminton Club	4407 Outlook Street, Madison, WI 53716	608/221-1887

GLOSSARY

Badminton Terms

Alley: The 1½-foot-wide area on each side of the court that is used for doubles.

Around-the-Head Stroke: An overhead stroke used when hitting a forehand-like overhead stroke which is on the backhand side of the body.

Back Alley: The area between the doubles' long service line and the back baseline.

Back Court: Approximately the back third of the court.

Backhand: A stroke made on the non-racket side of the body.

Base: *See* home base. Also the cork part of the shuttle in which the feathers are attached.

Baseline: The back boundary line of the court.

Bird: Another name for shuttlecock or shuttle.

Block: A soft shot, used primarily against a smash, in which there is little or no backswing or follow-through.

Carry: Called when the shuttle stays on the racket during a stroke. It is legal if the racket follows the intended line of flight. Also called *throw*.

Centerline: The line parallel with the sidelines, separating the service courts.

Clear: A high shot that goes over your opponent's head and lands close to the backline. Also called *lob*.

Combination Doubles Formation: Where the partners play both up and back and side by side.

Crosscourt: A shot hit diagonally into the opposite court.

Dab: A blocking action for a shot. Also called *push*.

Double Hit: An illegal shot in which the racket contacts the shuttle twice in one swing.

Doubles Service Court: The short, wide area (13 feet x 10 feet) to which the server must serve.

Down-the-Line Shot: A shot hit straight ahead—usually down the sideline.

Dribble: *See* hairpin drop.

Drive: A hard-driven stroke that clears the net but does not go high enough for your opponent to smash.

Drive Serve: A hard serve similar to the drive shot. It is used most often in doubles games, with a server serving from the right court to the backhand side of a right-handed player.

Drop: A shot that just clears the net, then falls close to it.

Face: The wide part of the racket—the part with the strings.

Fault: Any infraction of the rules. It results in the loss of serve or in a point for the server.

First Serve: A term used in doubles to indicate that the person serving is the first server of the inning.

Flick: A quick wrist action that speeds the flight of the shuttle.

Foot Fault: Called when the server's feet are out of the proper service court or when they leave the floor during a serve.

Forecourt: The area near the net—approximately between the net and the short service line.

Forehand: Any stroke made on the racket side of the body.

Game Point: The point that ends the game.

Hairpin Drop Shot: A soft shot made from close to the net and low, just clearing the net, then dropping nearly straight down.

Halfcourt Shot: A low shot that lands at approximately midcourt. It is used most often in doubles against teams playing in an up-and-back alignment.

Hand In: The term used to indicate that the server retains the serve.

Hand Out or One Hand Down: The term used in doubles when one player has lost service.

Home Base: The position in the center of the court from which the player can best play any shot hit by the opponent.

IBF: The International Badminton Federation—the world governing body.

Inning: The period of time during which a singles player or a doubles team is serving.

Kill: A fast, downward return, such as a smash, which should end the point.

Let: Called when play is stopped because of some outside interference. The point is then replayed.

Lob: *See* clear.

Long Serve: A high serve landing near the backline of the receiver.

Love: A term sometimes used to indicate that the score is zero.

Match: A series of games. The winner must win two out of three games or three out of five to win the match.

Match Point: The point that, if won, will win the game.

Midcourt: The middle third of the court, between the net and the baseline.

Net Shot: A shot executed in the forecourt that barely clears the top of the net.

Offense: The team or player that is hitting downward returns or forcing the opponent to lift the shuttle in the return.

Overhead: The arm action used to hit a shuttle when it is above one's head.

Placement: Controlling where a shot will land. Good placement directs a shot to an area of the court from which the opponent will find it difficult to make an effective return.

Pronation: The inward rotation of the wrist and forearm used for all overhead forehand strokes that require power.

Put the Bird on the Floor: End the rally with a kill or a well-hit placement where the opponents cannot get a racket on the bird.

Racket: The implement used to hit the shuttle.

Racket Foot: The foot on the racket side of the body. It will be forward on underhand strokes.

Rally: A period of hitting the shuttle back and forth over the net—either during practice or during a game.

Ready Position: The balanced position that a player assumes to be ready to move in any direction. The weight is on the balls of the feet, knees are bent, and the torso leans forward.

Receiver: The player to whom the shuttle is served.

Round the Head: *See* around-the-head shot.

Rush the Serve: A tactic used mostly in doubles by the receiver to quickly attack a low serve.

Scissors: The changing of position of the feet taken during a shot so that the hitter can get to the home-base area more quickly.

Second Serve: In doubles, the term indicates that one partner has lost the serve and the other partner is serving.

Server: The player who starts the play.

Set-Up: A shot that gives the opponent an easy chance to win the rally.

Setting: Making the choice as to how many more points to play when the score is tied one or two points before the game should be over—such as at 13 or 14 in a 15-point game.

Short Serve: A serve that clears the net low and lands just beyond the service line. It is used primarily in doubles play.

Shuttlecock or Shuttle: The feathered cork or plastic missile that is hit in the game of badminton.

Side By Side: A defensive formation used in doubles, in which each partner is responsible for one side of the court.

Side Out: When the individual or team loses the serve and the other team gets its chance to serve.

Smash: A hard overhead stroke hit sharply downward. It is the major attacking stroke in badminton.

Supination: The outward rotation of the wrist and forearm used for backhand strokes.

T: The intersection of the middle service and short service lines.

Underhand: The stroke used when the shuttle is hit below shoulder level.

Unsight: An illegal position taken by the server's partner so that the receiver cannot see the serve as it is hit.

Up and Back: An offensive formation used almost exclusively in mixed doubles, in which the front player is responsible for the forecourt and the partner for the backcourt.

Index

Alley 153
Around-the-head stroke 63–64, 153
Attacking clear service return 44
Attacking overhead clear shot 54

Back alley 153
Back court 153
Backhand grip 20–23
Backhand overhead clear stroke 54
Backhand serve 40–41
Backhand underhand clear 67–68
Back-scratching position 51
Badminton
  basics of 4
  benefits of 2
  drills 90–99
  equipment 6–10, 117
  history of 3
  increasing potential 102–111
  laws and courtesies of 12–17, 112–138
  self-tests 96–99
  strategy 74–88
  where to play 3
Badminton USA 139
Base 153, *See also* Home base
Baseline 153
Bird 7–8, 153
Block shot 68, 153

Carry 153
Centerline 153
Changing ends 118
Circular rotation alignment 80–81
Clear service return 43, 46, 153
Clothing 8
Combination doubles formation 153
Conditioning 104–111
  aerobic 110–111
  flexibility 108–110
  strength 104–108

Cooling down 31
Court 8–10, 113
Courtesies 12–13
Crosscourt 153

Dab service return 47
Dab shot 61, 153
Disabled players 128–130
Double hit 17, 153
Doubles drive service return 46–47
Doubles drop service return 44
Doubles service return 44–47
Down-the-line shot 85, 154
Dribble, *See* Hairpin drop shot
Drills 90–99
Drive serve 38–39, 154
Drive shot 61–63, 154
Drop shot
  overhead 59–60
  service return 44
  underhand 68

Equipment 6–10, 117

Face 7, 154
Fault 15–16, 121–122, 154
First serve 154
Flick serve 38, 154
Foot fault 154
Footwork 27–28
Forecourt 154
Forehand grip 20–23
Forehand overhead clear stroke 51–52
Forehand underhand clear stroke 66–67
Frying-pan grip 22

Game point 154
Goal setting 102

Grips 7, 20–23
    backhand 20–23
    forehand 20, 23
    frying pan 22

Hairpin drop shot (dribble) 69–71, 154
Halfcourt push service return 46
Halfcourt shot 154
Half-smash service return 44
Half-smash stroke 57–58
Hand in 154
Hand out 14, 154
High deep serve 34–36
Home base 24–25, 154
IBF 139
In 14
Inning 14, 154
International Badminton Federation (IBF) 139
Kill 155

Let 122–123, 155
Lob, *See* Clear
Long and short game 52
Long serve 155
Love 155

Match 155
Match point 155
Measurements 125
Mental practice 102–104
Midcourt 155

Net 113–115
Net shot 155
No set 14

Offense 155
Officials 124
    recommendations to 130–138
Onehand down, *See* Handout
Out 17
Overhead strokes 50–64
    around-the-head shot 63–64
    attacking clear 54
    backhand clear 54
    drive shot 61–63
    drop shot 59–60
    forehand clear 51–52
    half-smash 57–58
    push or dab shot 61
    smash 54–57
    throwing drill 53

Penalties 123–124
Placement 155
Posts 113
Practice
    conditioning 104–111
    drills 90–99
    mental 102–104
Pronation 155
Push shot, *See* Dab shot
Put the bird on the floor 75, 155

Racket 6–7, 117, 155
Racket foot 155
Raquet, *See* Racket
Rally 48, 155
Rally-ready position 23
Ready position 23–25, 155
    rally ready 23
    for return of service 23–24
Receiver 155
Relaxation 103–104
Round the head, *See* Around-the-head shot
Rules 13–17, 112–138
Rush the serve 156

Scissors 156
Scoring 118
Second serve 156
Serve 34–41, 118–121
    backhand 40–41
    drive 38–39
    flick 38
    high deep 34–36
    returning the 42–48
    short 36–38
Server 156
Service return 42–48
    attacking clear 44
    clear 43–46
    doubles 44–47
    doubles drive 46–47

    doubles drop 44
    drop 44
    halfcourt push 46
    half-smash 44
    push 47
    and scoring 47
    singles 42–44
    smash 44
Set-up 156
Setting 156
Shadow practice 27
Shoes 8
Short serve 36–38, 156
Shuttle 7–8, 116–117, 156
Shuttlecock 7–8, 116–117, 156
Side by side alignment 80–82, 85, 156
Side out 156
Singles service return 42–44
Smash service return 44
Smash stroke 54–57, 156
    deferring the 68–69
Socks 8
Strategy 74–88
    basic 74
    developing your 74
    doubles 79–85
    mixed doubles 85–87
    singles 74–78
Supination 156
Sweatbands 8
Switch step 64

T 85, 156
Throw, *See* Carry
Throwing drill 53
Toss 117
Tournaments 141–151
    the draw 142–148
    match scheduling 141–142
    operation of 149–151
    seeding the draw 144–146
Two hands down 15, 48

Underhand strokes 66–71, 156
    backhand underhand
        clear 67–68
    block shot 68
    defensing the smash 68–69
    forehand underhand clear 67–68
    hairpin drop (dribble) 69–71
    underhand drop 68
United States Badminton Association (USBA) 139–140
Unsight 156
Up and back alignment 80–85, 156
USBA 139–140

Visualization 102–103
Vocabulary 126–127

Warming up 28–31
Wedge formation 86–87